A PLUME BOOK

BODY WITH SOUL

RANDY JACKSON is a longtime music industry veteran and Grammy Award–winning rock bassist and record producer. He is also a member of the judging panel on *American Idol*, one of the most successful shows in the history of American television, and executive producer of the hit MTV series *Randy Jackson Presents: America's Best Dance Crew.*

BODY WITH SOUL

Shed Pounds, End Diabetes, and Transform Your Health

RANDY JACKSON

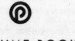

A PLUME BOOK

PLUME
Published by the Penguin Group
Penguin Group (USA) Inc., 375 Hudson Street, New York, New York 10014, USA •
Penguin Group (Canada), 90 Eglinton Avenue East, Suite 700, Toronto, Ontario M4P
2Y3, Canada (a division of Pearson Penguin Canada Inc.) • Penguin Books Ltd., 80
Strand, London WC2R 0RL, England • Penguin Ireland, 25 St. Stephen's Green, Dub-
lin 2, Ireland (a division of Penguin Books Ltd.) • Penguin Group (Australia), 250
Camberwell Road, Camberwell, Victoria 3124, Australia (a division of Pearson Aus-
tralia Group Pty. Ltd.) • Penguin Books India Pvt. Ltd., 11 Community Centre,
Panchsheel Park, New Delhi – 110 017, India • Penguin Group (NZ), 67 Apollo Drive,
Rosedale, North Shore 0632, New Zealand (a division of Pearson New Zealand Ltd.) •
Penguin Books (South Africa) (Pty.) Ltd., 24 Sturdee Avenue, Rosebank, Johannes-
burg 2196, South Africa

Penguin Books Ltd., Registered Offices: 80 Strand, London WC2R 0RL, England

Published by Plume, a member of Penguin Group (USA) Inc. Previously published in
a Hudson Street Press edition.

First Plume Printing, January 2010
10 9 8 7 6 5 4 3 2 1

Ⓟ REGISTERED TRADEMARK—MARCA REGISTRADA

The Library of Congress has catalogued the Hudson Street Press edition as follows:

Jackson, Randy.
  Body with soul : slash sugar, cut cholesterol, and get a jump on your best health
ever / Randy Jackson.
      p. cm.
  ISBN 978-1-59463-050-7 (hc.)
  ISBN 978-0-452-29565-0 (pbk.)
  1. Weight loss. I. Title.
  RM222.2.J28—2008
  613.2'5—dc22   2008030460

Printed in the United States of America

Penguin is committed to publishing works of quality and integrity.
In that spirit, we are proud to offer this book to our readers;
however, the story, the experiences, and the words
are the author's alone.

CONTENTS

This book is dedicated to all of the people who have struggled with weight loss and are continuing to do so in an effort to obtain optimal health. I love you! Continue the fight; we're all in this together. Keep hope alive and never forget that what you put into it is what you'll get out of it.

FOREWORD

Nearly two-thirds of adults and one-third of children in the United States are overweight or obese. There are 21 million Americans with diabetes; 54 million more have something called pre-diabetes, and most of them will develop diabetes if they don't change the way they live their lives. While it is easy for health care providers to simply tell people to change, those words do not enable people to magically lose weight and reduce their health risk. What is needed instead is for people to focus on the barriers that have kept them from losing weight in the past, to find an example to follow, and to put into place a plan that lasts a lifetime—not just a month or two. Randy Jackson's *Body with Soul* delivers on all those accounts. Randy takes the reader on his long odyssey, sharing what has worked for him and how it can be turned into success for others. In *Body with Soul*, Randy inspires, instructs, and instills the confidence needed to help people struggling with their weight find their own way to living a healthy lifestyle.

I met Randy in 2004, when he contacted me at Childrens Hospital Los Angeles to find out more about diabetes—and particularly the increase in type 2 diabetes, or what used to be called adult-onset diabetes, now occurring in record numbers of youth. He told me he was worried about our nation's children since so many had already developed unhealthy lifestyle habits and obesity. He was worried that children were starting to compile risk factors for cardiovascular disease, that they had sleep apnea, depression, risk for certain cancers, and stress on their joints and bones. He was concerned about the statement from authorities suggesting that this generation of Americans might not live as long as their parents and that one in three children born in the year 2000 and beyond will develop diabetes in their lifetimes if things don't change. Randy told me he knew from personal experience the diagnosis of diabetes was devastating, and that by the time someone developed diabetes it was almost too late. He told me in no uncertain terms that he wanted to do something, and to use his personal story and tremendous celebrity to make a difference. And that is exactly what he has done.

Randy immediately got involved with local childhood obesity prevention and treatment programs in Los Angeles; in fact, he helped secure funding for some of my own research in low-income neighborhoods in east and south Los Angeles. He worked at the national level as well, making video appearances to inspire youth to become more active and choose healthier foods. In each effort, he used himself as an example, an example of what went wrong, but how it's possible, even for an old dawg like him, to change. And in each instance, his message resonated with the youth he talked to who appreciated his honesty and sincerity.

Randy has written a phenomenal book. He lays out the simple truth: you can try fad diets and fancy exercise programs, you can spend a ton of money, and you can often succeed, but only for a limited amount of time, if that. Long-term success can only come when healthy habits become lifetime habits, when you make gradual changes that become the basis of how you live your life. Start small and build up over time. Add one good habit onto the next, and if you fall off the wagon, pick yourself up, dust yourself off, and get back on again. Learn moderation, and keep your eye on the ultimate reward: your own good health. And when you need to, just think of Randy and how, in the midst of temptation everywhere, he found the will to take control of his health and say no—to say no to obesity, to diabetes, and to suffering.

Randy has inspired me to get out there every day and make a difference, he has inspired the contestants on *American Idol* to give their best, and I know he can inspire you to do what you need to do to be a healthy, productive member of our world and live life to the fullest.

—Francine R. Kaufman, M.D.
Distinguished Professor of Pediatrics and Communications; The Keck School of Medicine and the Annenberg School of Communications of the University of Southern California; Head, Center for Diabetes, Endocrinology, and Metabolism, Childrens Hospital Los Angeles; Past President, the American Diabetes Association

INTRODUCTION

"**I** 'll meet you at the emergency room."

There are a few things you hope you'll never hear a doctor say, and *that* is definitely one of them. But there I was, on an otherwise uneventful day back in 1999, listening to those very same words over the phone. Actually, I was a little relieved. For five long days I had been feeling sick in the craziest kind of way—extremely tired, extremely thirsty, all sweaty and dizzy. It felt like I had a really bad cold or the flu, and although I had taken everything from aspirin to cold medicine to try and make myself feel better, nothing had helped. At least now I was going to find out what was wrong with me, even if it meant a trip to the hospital. "Let's see what's going on," said my doctor.

What was going on, it turned out, was diabetes.

My wife, Erika, and I drove over to the hospital and waited for my doctor to arrive. If you've ever been to the emergency room, you know it's a nasty place with all kinds of frightening stuff going on. In comparison with some of the casualties coming in—broken arms, bleeding heads—I thought my situation was pretty mild. I figured I'd breeze in and out of there, maybe with a prescription for antibiotics or something simple like that. When my doctor got to the hospital, Erika and I were whisked off to a room, and the nurses went to work, checking my blood pressure and sticking me with needles. My doctor had ordered a series of tests, including one that would determine the level of sugar in my blood. A short time later, I got the bad news. "It's kind of what I thought," my doctor told me. "You have type 2 diabetes. Your blood sugar is over 500."

To give you some idea of how scary that is, normal blood sugar readings are in the low hundreds. Mine was *five times* that. Damn, I had that "sugar." That's what they call diabetes where I come from: sugar. I could hear them now. "Boy, you got that sugar."

I shouldn't have been shocked to learn that I had diabetes, but I was. Yes, I was carrying about 350 pounds on my five-foot-eleven frame and both my parents had had the disease, two factors that put you at risk for type 2 diabetes. But these things always happen to somebody else, right? Even though, over the years, doctors had told me to watch it, to eat better and exercise more, I was really only listening to one voice—my own. And I was telling myself solely what I wanted to hear, which was that I was doing okay. I'd look in the mirror but not accept what I saw. "You're still hot!" I'd tell myself. But here's the reality: the route I was traveling on had a big, red, blinking sign by the side of the road, reading "Diabetes Ahead—Take the Detour!" Still, I just kept on driving in the same direction I always had.

There are certain words that can rock your world: I do. It's a girl. This is *American Idol*. You have diabetes. For me that last one has been both a blessing and a curse. It's a curse to be saddled with a disease that's life threatening and that you can't completely get rid of (though you can certainly manage it). But it's a blessing to get that huge wake-up call. After that day in the ER when my doctor burst the bubble I'd been living in, I couldn't lie to myself anymore. Right then and there I began my journey toward better health. I *had* to. It was a long journey, with lots of ups and downs, and it's not over yet—that's the thing you've got to understand, it's never over—but I have lost one hundred pounds and my diabetes is under control. I don't take any medication at all. And if I'm ever feeling fed up with the whole damn thing, all I've got to do is switch on *American Idol Rewind*, the show that recaps past seasons of *American Idol*. When I see my old self, I'm like, "Whoa, what was I thinking?!"

Maybe if I knew what was going on inside my body I would have acted faster, but diabetes creeps up on you. Like I said, I had two of the most obvious risk factors—being way overweight and having a family history of the disease—but I never really felt sick until that fatal week. Unless you're really in tune with your body, it's hard to know that your blood sugar is in the danger zone. A lot of people never figure it out until they, like me, end up in the emergency room. Statistics show that right now about one-third of the approximately 21 million Americans who have diabetes aren't even aware of it. That's a lot of "sugar" going undiagnosed.

Most people know me as a man on a mission to find the next American Idol. But after going through my own health scare, then dropping all those extra pounds, I've become a man on a mission to get Americans to improve their eating habits and get regular exercise. I established the Randy Jackson Childhood Obesity Foundation and signed on as a spokesman for the American Heart Association's Heart of Diabetes campaign, a drive to help people with type 2 diabetes manage the disease and understand its connection to cardiovascular disease (check it out: www.iknowdiabetes.org). If you can believe it, of the 21 million Americans who have diabetes, an estimated two-thirds of them will die of heart attack or stroke. Isn't that amazing? What's even more amazing is that more people probably know who Kelly Clarkson is than realize that diabetes is *connected* to cardiovascular disease and stroke. Having high blood sugar is destructive to the body in many ways, and one of those ways is that it causes fatty deposits to build up on the insides of the blood vessels. Those clogged vessels can then block the flow of blood to the heart, causing a heart attack, or to the brain, causing a stroke. Either way, it's a bad and potentially life-threatening deal.

What I want to do is help people who, like me, already have diabetes and also help people who are on the road to the disease or other weight-related diseases and health problems. If you are substantially overweight, there's a good chance that you are traveling in that direction. Yet by losing weight, eating more healthfully, and moving your body more, you can reverse course.

I want to spread the word that change, permanent change, is possible. I'm a new me, and I want you to be a new you. Even if you've had the same bad habits for ten, twenty, thirty years—I definitely did—you can get used to a healthier lifestyle. Old dawgs *can* learn new tricks. And you're talking to a dawg who tried everything in the past. Diets, liquid fasts, weight-loss medications, you name it, and none of them ever worked for long. But when I wound up in the hospital, I had to face up to why all those methods failed. Not to be overly dramatic, but it had really come down to a matter of life and death (or at least a life threatened by blindness, amputation, and the complications I mentioned earlier, heart disease and stroke). I had to figure out what would work for me, and ultimately I did. Now I want to tell you about it.

By telling you my story, I'm hoping to inspire you to put aside all the quick fixes and commit yourself to changing your lifestyle, because that, I know now, is what it takes to succeed. Whether you have two hundred, one hundred, or twenty-five pounds to lose, there is no diet or magic pill that's going to make you drop the weight you need to drop overnight. It's just not possible, so stop thinking about it. It's not going to happen. Instead, promise yourself that you're going to become healthy for the long run and not just lose weight because you're going to your high school reunion or because summer is coming and you want to go to the beach. Make a commitment. Put in the time. Put in the effort. Expect disheartening setbacks. Expect exhilarating breakthroughs. When it all works out in the end, you'll see that it was well worth it.

I believe that many things in life, while seemingly dissimilar, are really much the same. During the *Idol* season, the top ten finalists get up on that stage and give it their all. They don't just rely on their natural talent to garner votes. Instead, they present themselves each week with conviction, and they persevere, sometimes in the face of humiliating setbacks. (In season 7, for instance, Brooke White, David Archuleta, and Jason Castro all forgot lyrics at one point.) Mostly what they do, though, is work really hard, because they know that you've got to push yourself like crazy if you want to make it. The same thing goes for losing weight and improving your health—and really just about anything you do in life. Get in it to win it, baby, and you're going to succeed.

If you're like me, you've probably already read tons of books about weight loss. Here, though, is a book by a guy who knows what you're going through. I'm a big fan of self-help books, but I prefer the ones written by people who speak from experience. We can all use the help of doctors, fitness trainers, dietitians, psychologists, and other professionals, which is why I've asked several experts to contribute to this book. Their input is critical. But with all due respect to health gurus, most of them haven't had to lug around one hundred to two hundred extra pounds. Most of them don't know what it's like to find yourself in the emergency room because you ate too damn much for too damn long. Expert advice is essential, but to my mind it's also important to hear from people who have walked a mile in your shoes.

When you've got a lot of weight to lose, you're in an entirely different place than someone who just ate too much over the holidays. I used to hear people crying over the extra 20 pounds they gained when they got married or the 5 they put on while on vacation. Try telling that to someone who is 100 or 150 pounds overweight. Those people were having a fit, but I was *fat*. They had no idea what I was going through. That's why I always say, "Let me talk to the guy who broke his leg, not the guy who fixed the broken leg." This is a book about the problem of being overweight by a guy who was overweight for a long time—yet finally took control of his health.

There's a lot of conversation going on about obesity in this country. What I want to do is bring in the voice of someone who knows what it's like to be walking around with that extra hundred pounds. I'm the guy who has been on many of the diets recommended by skinny experts and who after a few weeks of doing everything right has woken up and said, "Hell, I don't want to do what someone else is telling me to do." I'm also the guy who, when he loses weight, hates to hear, "You look great!" Well, how did I look before? Like a water buffalo? Rebellion, tender feelings, and the overwhelming desire for foods we're not "supposed to" have—these are the things that overweight people constantly live with. Yet these things usually get left out of the mix in books written by people who haven't been there themselves.

In this book I'm going to be perfectly honest with you, even if it means saying some things you'd rather not hear. If you've ever watched *American Idol*, you know that I believe in telling it like it is. If a performance is just "awright for me, dawg," I'm going to say so. If it's "smokin' molten hot" or "pitchy," I'm going to say so too. So for starters, let's tell the truth about weight loss. Losing weight and keeping it off is hard: it's one of the hardest things you'll ever do. Even if you have a gastric bypass, which I did, and which I will tell you all about in chapter 4, it's still difficult. (Don't make the mistake of thinking that surgery is the easy way out.) But, oh my God, if you're able to win at losing, even come close to winning, you're way ahead of the game.

The rewards you get for your efforts are incredible: Losing just 5 to 10 percent of your body weight can lower your cholesterol, reduce your risk of getting type 2 diabetes by 60 percent, and improve your health substantially in several other ways. Just being able to shop in regular stores, to walk without your knees and back hurting, to get a good night's sleep (I am one of the many people who has had weight-related sleep apnea, a condition that makes it hard to breathe while you sleep) is a revelation. You're going to wonder why you didn't get busy earlier. And while you might think that looking better is the best reward, let me tell you, those other things are what make the effort worth it. And that's not even counting knowing you won't need insulin shots or other heavy-duty medications to get you through the day. We've all got busy, active lives to live, and knowing that we can live them without the challenge of carrying around extra weight is tremendous.

I don't think shedding pounds is easy for anybody, but it's particularly hard if you come from a culture that values not just eating but eating the most delicious sugar-, fat- and salt-drenched food *at every meal*. I come from *the* eating place, Baton Rouge, Louisiana—just an hour away from that other eating place, New Orleans—and when I was growing up, you didn't think twice about putting whatever you wanted into your mouth. The only stipulation was that everything had to taste unbelievable. It was all about being cooked to perfection and tasting good. If you saw a skinny chef in the South, you'd think, "That guy doesn't eat his own food! It must not be that good."

We didn't know from saturated fats or carbs or sugar. All

we knew was that there was always a reason to eat. Happy? Let's celebrate with food. Sad? There's food at the wake. After church there's eating. Before church there's eating. Birthday parties, weddings, holidays, Cousin Henry's back in town—there's eating. You eat together. You eat alone. And always something sinfully good, or what's the point?

This is how it is in the South, and while it's a little over the top—nobody knows how to eat like African American Southerners—it's really not all that different from how a lot of Americans eat. Even if an obsessive interest in food is not a typical part of your heritage or ethnic culture, much of life still revolves around eating: Let's have lunch. Let's go to dinner. Meet you for happy hour. Turn on the TV and you're hit with a million images of food. And most of the food that's out there? Come on! It kills—and not in the sense that a really great *Idol* contestant kills when she nails a song. I mean it literally kills.

Well, it kills some of us at least. That's the thing that's hard to accept: fat isn't fair. We all like to think that we can be as normal as the next person. I have a bunch of friends who are beanpoles, and they eat high-calorie food all the time—steak, fries, dessert, and four drinks at dinner—and they don't gain an ounce. I just watch them and go, "What? Why can't I do that? This isn't fair." And you know, it's not. But I've come to accept it, and you should too.

Anyway, it's like comparing apples and oranges—you're never going to win if you compare yourself to someone whose DNA is completely different from yours. If there is one thing I have learned on this journey, it's that I've got to deal with my own body and my own circumstances and quit wishing that I had the metabolism of someone else. Don't judge Peter by looking at Paul and Mary over there. It's never going to add up.

I often tell aspiring singers to stay in their own lane. Just like a horse in the Kentucky Derby wearing blinders, you can't be concerned with what anyone else is doing or what genetic gifts they've got. Deal with you. Don't worry about the guy over there doing red-hot ballads when you are better at doing a Blake Lewis beatbox thing. Don't think about getting a sculpted 2-percent-body-fat body like Madonna's when destiny has handed you a more rounded (but curvy and sexy!) shape. Keep those blinders on.

I would love to be a racecar driver or an airplane pilot, but I've accepted that there are certain things I can't do. A lot of us have grown up with the ideology that you can be whatever you want to be if you just put your mind to it. Well, yes, in some respects. I certainly put my mind to being a musician, and here I am, thanks to a combination of hard work and natural talent. But only some things are within our reach, no matter how hard we try. And for most people, including me, a movie-star body isn't one of them.

When you think about it, it's kind of funny that I ended up on a reality show, because I try to live my life in cold, hard reality. And the reality is that much as I may want my body to be what society considers perfect, it's never going to be like that. But just the same, my body can be healthy and I can feel good about it—which I do!

It took me many years of fruitless diets, culminating in a giant health crisis, to come to this conclusion. But I eventually discovered that if I stopped trying to be perfect, I would have greater success at losing weight. Along the way I also had a few other epiphanies that helped me shed pounds and keep them off for what's now been five years. Some of those revelations had to do with learning how to get used to eating less and exercising more, which of course is the crux of the matter. But what I found to be even more essential were the eureka moments that changed the way I *think* about weight loss. After being diagnosed with diabetes, I approached weight loss with a different attitude, and it made all the difference in the world.

First, and most important, I realized that I had to lose weight for me and me alone. I couldn't do it because some groovy people thought it was uncool to be fat or even because my family was worried about me. The motivation had to be that I cared enough about myself to do what I had to do.

Look, it's not easy to ignore the pressure society puts on people to be thin and instead to focus on asking yourself what *you* need. I know this firsthand. My pre-*Idol* career as a bass player, music producer, and record company executive took me all over the world, with stints living in New York, San Francisco, Houston, and finally Los Angeles, where I now hang my hat. This is the town where everyone, by reputation at least, is thin, beautiful, living on fat-free tacos, and working out like a maniac. So just walking down the street, I was different. Then there was *American Idol*. Every week millions of people were looking at me sitting beside slender Paula and taking hits from Simon. ("It looks like you're wearing Randy's pants!" he once said to an oversized Idol wannabe.) I even had the odd pissed-off contestant call me "fat" as a zillion viewers looked on. ("No kidding," I said to him. "Are you sure?")

Introduction

I've been in the entertainment business for a long time, so I'm used to being judged. I *am* a judge, and I firmly believe that if you're going to dish it out, you've got to be able to take it too. But that isn't to say I was completely immune to the pressure. And then there was my family. I have a beautiful wife and three fantastic kids that I want to be there for—my daughters, eighteen-year-old Taylor and twelve-year-old Zoe, and my ten-year-old son, Jordan. When I was diagnosed with diabetes, Erika was scared, and of course she wanted me to get it together. But despite that, I didn't really take the steps I needed to take to lose weight until I realized that *I* wanted to get control over my health. I wanted it for me.

Losing weight and getting healthy is not a decision that anyone else can make for you. Your doctor, your significant other, your mother, brother, sister, uncle—it doesn't matter who it is. They can all want it for you, but you really have to want it for yourself. While it's great if they all support you and will help you in whatever ways they can, dropping pounds is a personal struggle. You have to want it for yourself, and ultimately you have to do it alone. Nobody is going to force you to get on a treadmill or follow you around making sure that you don't have Milky Way bars stashed in your desk drawer. It's all about you.

The other important revelation that came to me after my diabetes diagnosis is that to reach your goals you have to have patience. Nobody ever tells you that. Instead, they're all giving you timelines: lose ten pounds in ten days and so on. But think about this for a minute: you are trying to undo years and years of damage and bad eating habits. It takes time, first to change those habits in such a way that you can stick with the new, healthier ones, and then to actually drop the pounds. And this is true even if you have a gastric bypass.

Weight-loss surgery might seem like the ultimate quick fix, but it's not. For me it was just a jump start—a way to feel better and get motivated to do the work I had to do to keep the weight off. With a gastric bypass, you may drop eighty pounds right away, but that next twenty, forty, or sixty pounds can take months and years. And it's not like you can just sit back during that time and watch the fat fall off. You have to practice healthy eating and exercise habits, same as anyone who didn't have the surgery. Working up to the point where those habits are ingrained takes time. If ever patience was a virtue, it's going to be when you start out on this road.

Another thing that's absolutely essential is moderation. You've probably heard that before, and maybe you're sick and tired of hearing it. What could be more boring than moderation? But if I can embrace moderation, I'm telling you that you can too. I was barely out of college when I began my life as a full-time professional musician, so by the time my health hit bottom I had been living the rock-and-roll life for years. And the rock-and-roll life is not about moderation—it's the antithesis of moderation. So you can see that even including the word in my vocabulary was a big leap. But I'm a convert! I am now Mr. Moderation, and I believe it's the key to a great life. I don't care whether it's sex, drugs, drinking, food, exercise, or whatever, moderation really works, and in most cases it works better than perfection.

Maybe you're thinking you'd like to strive for total self-discipline: "Randy, I'm never going to eat chocolate again!" But you can't tell me that giving up something completely isn't just going to make you want it all that much more. It's human nature. If there's one thing I learned from all those diets I tried throughout the years, it's that taking all the pleasure out of eating is a surefire way to end up fat all over again. Same thing if you go overboard with exercise. I know people who've worked out like fiends and then crashed and burned. I'll run into them and they've put on thirty pounds because they just got tired of working out.

Going to extremes, especially trying to maintain a diet that gives you absolutely no pleasure whatsoever, tends to set you up for failure. It's the rare person who can go from excessive indulgence to zero indulgence and not go crazy. Before you know it, you're at the doughnut shop around the corner, buying the baker's dozen. But a morsel of something delicious here and there, that's not going to tip you over the edge. Moderation, I'm telling you—it's the way to go.

This book is all about living moderately while still living well. I'm not going to tell you that I eat the perfect textbook diet every day. I still go out to restaurants, I eat delicious food, and I even have sweets now and then. (It's a myth that diabetics can't eat any sugar at all.) Some days I do better than others. But I've figured out what works for me. I know that the way I eat now helped me drop enough weight to get my diabetes under control and to set a good example for my children. I'm all for striving for perfection in your professional life, but when it comes to eating, your mission (should you choose to accept it) is to get healthy within your own parameters. My credo is "I don't want to be perfect . . . just pretty good."

My grandma used to say, "There's no Christ walking the planet," and no matter what your religious beliefs are you know what she was talking about: nobody's perfect. If there are thirty-one days in a month and I eat right on twenty-five of them, I feel as though I'm doing okay. Diets often ask you to be perfect, which is another reason I don't like them. Same with some of these grandiose exercise programs. If you don't run five miles a day and lift weights four times a week, you feel pretty bad about yourself. That's just counterproductive. My attitude is to try to be the best that *I* can be.

I also believe that everyone has to find his or her own way of losing weight. Maybe the eating and exercise strategies that have worked for me will work for you too; that's why I've collaborated with the experts mentioned earlier (more on them in a few pages) to include a fourteen-day meal plan, recipes to go with it, and exercise advice in this book. But even if my strategies don't fit you to a T, at the very least this information will give you a place to start. The meal plan reflects my philosophy of allowing yourself small indulgences so that weight loss isn't such a punishing process. It's not a diet in the sense that you go on it, then take a hiatus once you've lost weight. Rather, it's a way of eating— but let me add, a *reasonable* way of eating—that you'll need to stick to permanently if you hope to get rid of those pounds and keep them off. (By the way, you're going to totally dig the nutritious, low-calorie, mostly Southern recipes the chef Jeff Parker, created for the meal plan and that run throughout the book. Even a Baton Rouge boy like me can hardly tell that they've been slimmed down. Shrimp and sausage gumbo ya ya, Cajun meat loaf, sweet potato pie, and more—they taste like the real deal.)

If you're the kind of person who needs guidelines, both the eating plan and the exercise section of this book will help you make the transition to healthier living. Maybe you need to drop a hundred pounds and, like me, have struggled with your weight for years. Maybe you're just noticing that your pants no longer fit, and you want to nip weight gain in the bud before it begins to take a toll on your well-being. It doesn't matter if you're an old hand at the diet game or have never tried to lose weight before, the strategies I'm offering can point you in the right direction. Ultimately, though, I fully expect that you'll tailor the program to your own specific needs. To really succeed, you've got to find ways of eating and exercising that jibe with your likes, dislikes, and lifestyle. Otherwise it's like following the grapefruit diet when you hate grapefruit—there's no way you're going to stay with it.

Everybody knows what it takes to lose weight; why they don't do it is the question. I think it's because most people don't take into consideration what works for them as individuals, what's *realistic* for them. They're always jumping on the latest diet bandwagon or trying out the newest exercise trend without thinking about how it suits their own life. Are you really going to be able to stay on a diet that requires that you bring your lunch every day and always eat dinner at home? Not me. I've got business meals practically every day of the week. Are you really going to go to the gym after work when you know your kids are waiting for you to get home and help them with their homework? Get real.

In this book I ask you to consider your life—not to change it but to consider it—and look for the ways you can work more exercise and healthier eating into your days and nights. I knew I wasn't going to turn my personal and professional life upside down just to accommodate more healthful choices, and I found I didn't have to.

Just like in every other aspect of life, losing weight requires being true to yourself. It's not all that different from what goes on during *American Idol* each season. It may seem like Simon, Paula, and I simply pass judgment on a performance: was it good or was it bad? But it's more than that. We're also trying to help singers learn what kind of music is right for them, so that when they perform they have a genuine connection to the song. If they aren't authentic, you can feel it right down to your toes. They don't sing well. Nothing gels. Before *Idol*, when I was an executive signing acts for record companies, my line to artists was, "If you don't know who you are, and I don't know who you are, then record buyers are not going to care who you are."

So being yourself is paramount. But while I've always known this from my work as a musician, I only understood recently that the same rules apply to how I approach my health as well. What I learned is that great success comes when you keep it real, find your own unique path to good health, and stay on it.

Above all, I want you to read this book and say to yourself, "I can do that." Everything I suggest is based on real-life circumstances, not an idealized world where there are no temptations or sticky situations that make it hard to be active and eat right. I know you're going to walk into Starbucks one day and see that piece of cake staring back at you from the display case.

Who's Who: A Little Help From the Experts

No man is an island, and I'm certainly not, especially when it comes to offering health advice. I talked to several knowledgeable people while preparing to write this book, and you'll find their words of wisdom mingled with my own observations and experiences throughout these pages. Here are some of the professionals you're going to meet:

Erin Naimi, RD

Erin is a registered dietitian in private practice. She has had considerable experience working with gastric bypass patients at Cedars-Sinai Medical Center in Los Angeles and at eating-disorder treatment centers. What I like most about Erin is her reasonable approach to nutrition. She, like me, doesn't believe in diets or deprivation. Rather, she's a fan of regulating your eating by learning to listen to your body's hunger signals. You'll hear a lot more about that in chapter 5.

Janeen Locker, PhD

Dr. Locker has treated people at Yale University and UCLA Neuropsychiatric Institute as well as at a leading eating-disorder treatment center in Southern California. Now in private practice in Santa Monica, California, she spends a lot of time helping patients who battle weight-related issues.

I wanted to get Dr. Locker's take on weight loss because I don't think you can separate the way you eat from the way you think about food and your body.

Tarik Tyler
Tarik is an in-demand, high-energy personal trainer in Hollywood, known for keeping his clients motivated. You're probably thinking, "Oh, he wants me to 'train' like a movie star now." I know that the very word *trainer* makes it sound like there is torture coming your way! Not at all. I think walking, simple walking, is the best exercise, and Tarik has some tips, starting in chapter 7, on how to maximize its health-promoting effects.

If you're up for a bigger challenge, we have some other exercise options to offer you too. None of them require turning into a gym rat (in fact, none of them require going to the gym at all). This is exercise for real people with busy lives. I've also created some playlists of music to listen to as you go. It's easy to forget you're working out when you've got a soulful voice singing in your ear.

Brittania Erickson
A great athlete and former softball player who now trains adults and teaches fitness to kids, Brittania has a very creative approach to exercise. If you're up for kicking your physical activity up a notch, she's got a great recipe for keeping it interesting.

Catherine Chiarelli

A dancer, singer, actress, trainer, and fitness-class instructor, Catherine has a lot to say about getting energized for exercise. Part of losing weight is really getting in touch with your body and making it feel good. Catherine's tips will help you ease into physical activity.

I know you're going to stop at a fast-food restaurant en route to your summer vacation. I know your boss isn't going to take too kindly to the idea of you skipping out early because you need to meet up with your walking partner. So what choices are you going to make? Helping you make the right ones is what I'm going for here.

As you read about my journey from 350-pound guy with sky-high blood sugar to dude that's got it all under control, some of it may seem disconcertingly familiar. The eating jags. The dieting penance. Dealing with the need to reverse behaviors ingrained in you (and often sanctioned by well-meaning grandmas!) from day one. Even if our lives are hugely different—maybe you don't hail from the South and have never laid a finger on a musical instrument—we've undoubtedly faced many of the same challenges. I hope that by seeing yourself in these pages, you'll also see yourself in its conclusion—a new, healthier you. I think you'll be surprised at how making a few small changes can get pounds to drop off and appreciably improve your health-indicator numbers. It's a great feeling to get your lab workup back and see that you've lowered your blood sugar, bad cholesterol, and triglycerides while raising your heart-protective good cholesterol.

To reach that point, you can't hold back. You've got to plunge in and change your habits. But take that dive from a sturdy platform. That's what the eating and exercise strategies in this book are, a platform, a jumping-off point for a new you. They're not designed to be some masochistic test of your willpower and fortitude. Remember, you will never be immune to temptation, but by learning to listen to your body's signals you can stop yourself from overeating and considerably reduce how much of the "wrong thing" you end up consuming. I'm hoping that the collection of reasonable ideas that follow will help you think differently about getting healthy. There is a lot here to help you.

The day I found out I had diabetes was pivotal for me, but it shouldn't have taken that dire diagnosis to clue me in to the fact that I have a disease. And when I say I have a disease, I'm not talking about the diabetes. In a way, being overweight is itself a disease, or at least that's how I think we should look at it. Most of us who are very overweight have been dealt a genetic card that mandates that we live differently from all those skinny guys with NASCAR-quick metabolisms. It's not fair, but it's real.

I tried and tried to lose weight for many years; I bet many of you have too. I found that success comes when you turn that corner and leave your old habits behind. Not your old *self*—you have got to be you—but I believe it's possible to change the way you're living your life without losing your heart and soul. I did it, and I know you can too!

Living differently, though, doesn't mean living unhappily.

There's a happy medium between following some bleak, wacky diet and eating like there's no tomorrow. I've found that place, and now I want to help you get there. You've got a shot to be the best you can be in this life, so go for it. And do it for the right reason: your health. When you do, nothing's going to stop you. You'll be living life in perfect pitch.

A Word About the Recipes

The recipes you'll find throughout the book are primarily Southern in flavor, yet with none of the blood-sugar-raising, artery-clogging characteristics that typify Southern food. All the dishes are the handiwork of Jeff Parker, a chef known for his high-quality, low-calorie food. Jeff has worked as a personal chef and develops recipes for the Food Network. Each of his recipes is incredibly easy to make, and he has also provided notes on the major utensils and pans you'll need (that way there's no working halfway through a recipe only to find that you don't have the nine-by-thirteen-inch pan you need). He also includes modifications for those of you watching your sodium intake. But with or without the added salt, you're going to love them. Dig in!

BODY WITH SOUL

CHAPTER ONE

The King Cake Chronicles

Take some flour, a mess of eggs, a big chunk of butter, plenty of sugar and cinnamon, mix it up, shape it into a ring, then fill the whole thing with something incredibly sinful like coconut cream cheese, chocolate bourbon pecan, praline, or cookies and cream. If you're feeling it, throw in some M&M's and raisins, bake it, ice the top, and cover it with three types of colored sugar. You now have what's known as a Mardi Gras King Cake, one of the most delectable and decadent pastries you can get your mouth on. It's like nine cakes in one.

When I think of the way I grew up eating, I think of the King Cake because it's a perfect representation of how eating and tradition come together in the South. It comes from a French ritual of baking a cake to honor the three kings who came bearing gifts to the baby Jesus twelve days after his birth—Twelfth Night. Louisianans adopted the tradition of the King Cake in celebration of carnival, which begins on Twelfth Night and ends with Mardi Gras (the day before Ash Wednesday, leading up to Lent).

Mardi Gras in Louisiana, and especially New Orleans, is one raucous event. It's days of nonstop parties and parades, with participants donning the wildest, most creative costumes you've ever seen. And all this has been going on since the 1830s. Mardi Gras is an enduring tradition; not even Hurricane Katrina stopped it from happening (thought it did curtail the festivities).

Now Mardi Gras wouldn't be Mardi Gras without the King Cake (Mardi Gras does, after all, translate into "Fat Tuesday"). The cake is decorated with tinted sugars representing the colors of Mardi Gras: gold for power, green for faith, and purple for justice. Hidden inside is a tiny plastic baby. Find that baby, and you've got the privilege (or the burden, depending on how you look at it) of throwing the next King Cake party.

I wouldn't quite say that life is always a party in Louisiana, especially during these post-hurricane days, but when I was a kid, you ate like you were celebrating. Some families might not have been able to buy this or that, but food was cheap, so you could always put something fantastic on the table. There was constant encouragement to eat. "My God, you're looking like skin and bones," my grandmother would say. "You better eat something." In my Southern, African American world, just like in a lot of cultures that struggled with adversity in the past, being able to eat as much and whatever you wanted was a sign of prosperity. The inevitable pounds that came with that were considered a good sign too.

Once, when I was in the beginning of my career—and the beginning of what would become a twenty-five-year struggle with weight—I returned home for a visit. Our family minister took one look at me and said, "Man, you've put on some weight. You must be living good!" Nowadays, even in the South, where they're finally getting worried about obesity, someone might say that sarcastically. "Man, you've been living *too* good" is what they'd really mean. But back then it was a compliment and, if not exactly encouragement, one of the many things that I felt gave me license to keep overeating.

Where the Fat Is

It's a good thing I'm not a betting man. I would never have picked Las Vegas as the fattest city in the nation, but that's what *Men's Fitness* magazine found in its 2008 survey. Guess it must be all those buffets: "All you can eat for $2.49!" "Eighteen hundred pancakes for $1.99!" I would have guessed that the fattest city is in the South, and while I didn't get it right, I wasn't all that far off the mark. Seven out of the top ten cities were pretty far south: five in Texas, one in Oklahoma, and one in Florida.

Some other statistics point to the fact that when you look at states rather than cities, the South has an obesity problem. As does the whole country. A group called the Trust for America's Health did a survey in 2007 and found that obesity rates in thirty-one states jumped from the previous year. Sadly, no states experienced a decrease. That doesn't surprise me. When we go out to cities around the country for preliminary *American Idol* auditions, I see this country's obesity problems firsthand. New York. Dallas. New Orleans. Kansas City. Miami. Chicago. Boston. But to tell the truth, I don't even have to leave California to see that there is a problem. It's everywhere across the state, even (though perhaps less apparent) right here in Hollywood.

Believe me, I'm not trying to slam my beloved home region, the South, but things are looking particularly bad down there. At 30 percent, Mississippi has one of the highest obesity rates in the country (Colorado has the lowest, with just over 17 percent). The state I grew up in, Louisiana, ranked fifth most obese in the country. That's just sad, but I'm not all that surprised. Walk down the aisle in a Southern grocery store and you'll see a smorgasbord of sweets and an ungodly amount of other kinds of edible junk—potato chips in seven flavors, fifteen kinds of snack cakes and pies—that you won't find anywhere else in the country. Southerners, we've got to get it together!

Most of the eating habits that eventually caused my weight to balloon to 350-plus pounds were ingrained in me from an early age. In my family, as in many of my Southern neighbors' families, every meal was a joyful celebration of life. You just didn't sit down to eat without an extravaganza of feel-good foods coming at you. My father, Herman, an oil company plant foreman, had thirteen brothers and sisters; my mother, Julia, had six; and not one of them was a slouch when it came to turning out golden fried chicken, mashed potatoes with cream gravy, and our Louisiana specialty, red beans and rice. My mother taught kindergarten for a while, but she also was a professional baker, famous for her homemade doughnuts and cinnamon rolls. My granny was known for her signature sweet potato pie (with its flaky lard crust). These weren't just treats that we had once in a while on special occasions. *We had them all the time.*

There were five of us in my immediate family: Mom, Dad, my brother, sister, and me—the baby. Life revolved around eating, work, church, and family. On Sundays you'd come home from church and have a huge spread. Not a couple of pieces of toast, but grits, eggs, bacon, bread, pancakes, and all doused with butter.

We'd sit down to dinner every night and have a pretty big meal. It might be something like fried chicken or meat loaf. There were always several courses, and we never ate anything green without plenty of fatback, bacon, or butter to give it flavor. We didn't just have corn, we had creamed corn with bacon bits in it. We also always had bread or corn bread, potatoes or rice. There was a lot of starch. Desserts were consistently a part of the meal too, and I'm not talking about a cup of strawberries. It was a sacrilege to serve anything other than a proper dessert like scoops of homemade butter pecan ice cream slapped on top of a fresh-baked pecan pie. At the end, we'd pat our bellies. Mmm, that was good. Eating was always supposed to be really delicious. No one understood why you'd eat something if it wasn't great. *What do you mean, eating for health reasons? What do you mean, I need more fiber? If it doesn't taste good, I'm not eating it.*

And that was just the meals. The snacks were outrageous too. Grape Nehi sodas, Stage Plank gingerbread cookies (once called Rock 'n' Roll cookies, which, not surprisingly, I totally dug), raisin pies with cream in the middle, huge cinnamon rolls with blobs of icing and big enough for two or three people (but usually eaten by one), dozens of doughnuts still so hot from the oil that you could squish them together till they looked like just one or two. Ice cream sundaes, ice cream cones, MoonPies, and RC Cola. Praline pecan candy made with pounds of butter, sugar, pecans, and condensed milk. Anything sweet and gooey was golden in my eyes. Whatever it was, maybe you'd have it with a glass of milk to make yourself feel a little more conscientious, but for the most part no one ever thought about health. We didn't know from trans fats or any of that. Let me amend that. We thought we were eating healthfully, in a way. As one of my uncles used to say, "If it's good *to* you, you know it's good *for* you."

If I had to single out one dish as my favorite from those days, it would be gumbo. It's almost a mystery dish because there's just so much stuff in it: sausage, chicken, pork, okra, beans. What do you want? Throw it in there. And calories? The flour-fat base of the stew, called a roux, alone could be 1,000 calories per bowl depending on who's making it. It's absolutely delicious. Crawfish étouffée (*étouffée* is French for "smothered," so you know it was something good), all that Creole Southern cooking was just fantastic. If you've ever watched *Emeril Live* you know what I'm talking about, but back in the day the big chef, and I mean that in more ways than one, was Paul Prudhomme, who really made Cajun cooking famous. He is this large, robust guy, and he had these barbecued ribs smothered in sauce made with bacon, honey, and dry-roasted pecans that were just, *woo!* They were good.

In the South of my youth, taste was everything, and the first forkful of food had to be as delicious as the last. If you had to put salt and pepper on the table, whoever was doing the cooking hadn't been doing his job right. Food was so important that you didn't go out with a girl unless she could bake and burn (cook). If she couldn't burn, what are you going out with that girl for? For us it was true that the way to a man's heart is through his stomach. Everywhere I lived after Baton Rouge—Houston, New York, LA, San Francisco—I'd test the waters by asking about food. "Does anyone here bake?" If the girls didn't bake, I'd be, like, "These are not real girls. Don't cook, don't bake. Something's wrong here." My wife? Yeah, she can burn a little.

Real-Life Alert
Making It Through the Holidays

The holidays—don't those two words just strike fear in your little heart? When you're trying to lose weight, it's hard not to dread them. It's always been tough for me because of how I grew up. I've been telling you about how over the top eating was back then, but that was just the everyday. You should have seen the Christmas and Thanksgiving holidays! Think andouille sausage and grits, jambalaya, bread pudding with bourbon sauce, beignets—then double that. It was outrageous. Even if the holidays are a little more subdued here in LA, I still get tempted by the fixin's, just like everybody else. But I've got a trick or two up my sleeve now that help me get through the seasonal festivities—and, for that matter, any party, any time of year.

First, let's talk about what not to do. I used to employ a strategy that I think a lot of people use: starve yourself all day so that you can cash in your calorie allowance at the big Thanksgiving dinner or the office Christmas party. It seems reasonable, but it tends to backfire. By being "good" during the day, you're likely giving yourself license to be "bad" at night, which means that you are going to go wild once you hit that holiday bar and buffet. You're going to be so hungry that nothing will be off limits. At the end of the evening you'll have racked up a ton of calories.

Here's a better approach, advocated by registered dietitian Erin Naimi. Eat normally throughout the day, then go to the party feeling appropriately hungry—not ravenous. Look at what's being offered, and allow yourself three or four things that you really love. You might, for instance, forget about having the bread *and* the stuffing and just have the stuffing instead. Don't have the sweet potatoes *and* the mashed potatoes; again choose between them (the sweet potatoes). Forgo a piece of pecan pie *and* a piece of pumpkin pie; have just a small slice of the pecan instead (or if both are absolutely irresistible, a few bites of each). I fully subscribe to the "morsel diet"—a morsel of this and a morsel of that isn't going to hurt you.

I don't know about you, but I remember some of those holiday meals where I ate so many different dishes that I hardly tasted any of them. "Choosing three or four dishes instead of, say, seven lets you really appreciate them, savor them, and be truer to how hungry you're really feeling," says Erin. I agree. It's easier for me to stop when I'm not in a mad rush to get in a million foods for fear that I won't see them for another year. This is the happy medium I'm always talking about. I get to eat some of those special holiday foods, but I don't leave the party feeling angry at myself (and sick to my stomach) for overeating.

It's easy to look back on those years and ask, "What were we thinking, eating that way?" Maybe it's true what they say: ignorance *is* bliss. I didn't know how destructive my eating habits were. But it was also a fine time in my life. Being with your family, enjoying food. There's nothing better. Now, of course, I know that you can do the same thing without upping the chance that you're going to have a heart attack later in the day. At the time, though, we were just doing what a lot of American families did and still do: celebrating being together with really good food.

The other day I was talking to a friend who is also from the South, and we agreed that the best thing about all that eating was what it represented—it was all about family and community. If you could sit down and eat with someone, then that person was all right. But the greatest thing about this tradition is also one of the deadliest things about it. It gets you into the habit of complete and utter indulgence. You don't want to eat anything unless it's got all that sugar and fat going on, and we all know where that eventually gets you. We're all products of the food-related rituals and attitudes instilled in us when we were young.

A friend said to me the other day, "Peanut butter and jelly sandwiches just don't taste the same when they're on whole wheat bread." This guy grew up eating PB and J on white bread; to him that combination, with its unique texture and feel, is home. This is the kind of thing you're up against when you decide that you need to change. So it's hard. Food not only gets our taste buds excited because it tastes good, it also evokes memories and provides comfort. That's just part of being human and not something I think we should entirely remove from our lives.

My experience has been that when you do cut out all pleasure and comfort from your eating life, you end up right back where you started. I'm sure no one really loves fat-free anything. If I blindfolded you and gave you two cookies, one fat free, one with fat, you'd prefer the one with fat. It's a no-brainer. But there is a middle ground. The challenge is to find that happy medium where you can eat healthfully without completely forsaking all the pleasures of good food.

As a kid, I never thought about finding the happy medium, and, the truth is, I didn't really seem to need to. I was outside playing all day long. All the kids in my hood were. We ran around; played football, basketball, and horseshoes; rode our bikes for miles. We were out and about at all times. We didn't think of it as exercise. Nobody in those days did, neither kids nor parents. In my hood, adults didn't belong to gyms and they didn't engage in formal exercise. Part of that was the era—my youth took place somewhat before the big gym-going craze started—and part was due to economics and culture (we weren't exactly golf club members). There wasn't a consciousness about physical activity the way there was in some segments of society.

So as a kid, I didn't know what *exercise* meant, but I did know how to have fun. Unfortunately, it's not that way for most kids anymore. With unsafe neighborhoods and playgrounds that are either nonexistent or commandeered by gangs, it's tough for kids to get out and move.

I was a big-boned kid but I wasn't fat, and that was probably because I was so active. Besides just running around with my friends, I was involved in competitive sports, both track and football. I was also playing music early on, but it wasn't yet my focus. Sports were where I was spending most of my time. In high school I was a shot put and discus man, and I played middle linebacker, guard, and tackle for our football team—I moved around a lot.

I suspect that this natural inclination to wear a lot of hats, developed early in my life, has served me well as an *Idol* judge. Once in a while, Simon, Paula, and I will get flack from some indignant "fans" who want to know what qualifies us to be so certain about a singer's performance and his or her chances of making it as a star. This is where I like to throw out my peripatetic professional life as proof that I know what I'm talking about. We all have years and years of experience: Simon as a record company executive, Paula as a much-in-demand choreographer and pop singer, and me as a journeyman (and Journey man) musician, producer of records, record industry executive, and radio host (*Randy Jackson's Hit List*, a syndicated show on Sunday mornings).

From those various vantage points, I've been able to get a good sense of what works and what doesn't. Are we always 100 percent right about who's going to make it and who's not? No, but we have a pretty good track record. One thing fans have to remember is that we are judging performances individually. How did we let someone like Jennifer Hudson, now an Academy Award winner, slip away? We judged her on the performances she gave at the time, not on her overall talent, which is of course remarkable. There are a lot of factors that go into choosing an American Idol (and, actually, *we* don't choose the Idol, America does).

Okay, now where was I? (Kind of got off on a tangent there, didn't I?) Oh yes, sports. Before I really got serious with the bass, sports were just the bomb to me. During this highly athletic time in my life, I paid a little more attention to nutrition than usual. You have to: you're dealing with endurance and conditioning. But I was also working out so much that I was burning off all those slices of sweet potato pie and heaps of greens cooked in fatback. And if you're working out three to four hours a day, I don't care what you eat, you're going to keep the weight off. Those hours—plus the time you're sleeping (and you need the extra sleep if you're going at it hard)—are also hours that you don't spend snacking, so that helps keep your body leaner too. Remember, calories in, calories out.

Football: A Double-Edged Sword

Football was good to me. There's nothing like being part of a team to teach kids how to work together, sacrifice, and look out for one another. Playing on my high school team also kept me active. Football practice wasn't exercise in the punishing sense of the word; it was just fun, plain and simple.

I think it's great for kids to be involved in sports, and I'm so glad that football was part of my life. But here's something about the game that I think is pretty interesting. Researchers have been looking at the correlation between obesity and youth football, and their findings have not been positive. One study published in the *Journal of the American Medical Association* found that 45 percent of high school linemen were overweight. Of those, 9 percent could even be considered severely obese. And they looked at a lot of kids—over thirty-five hundred. Another study had similar findings. This one, from the *Journal of Pediatrics,* also showed that 45 percent of the kids were overweight. And these kids were only ages nine to fourteen. That's really young to be battling so much weight.

Was I overweight when I played football? I was big, no doubt about it, and maybe, looking back, I was *too* big. There is a lot of pressure on football players (and not just in high school) to be oversized. It's part of the game, but it also gives some kids an excuse for being overweight. I'm hoping, though, that coaches are clueing in to the dangers of pressuring kids to put on more weight than is healthy.

If you've got a young football player at home, check it out: don't confuse big with healthy. And don't assume that the reason he is big is because he plays football. People would say to me, "Wow, you're a big kid; you must be playing football." It's like saying to someone, "You're tall; you must be a basketball player." All those assumptions don't make being big healthy. Don't let your kid jeopardize his well-being just to play the game.

Shrimp and Sausage Gumbo Ya Ya

I was surprised at how simple this gumbo recipe is, and Chef Jeff uses a clever trick—baking the flour in the oven—that allows you to avoid making a high-calorie roux.
Serves 12

Have on hand:
baking sheet
medium bowl
large, heavy straight-sided skillet or Dutch oven

3/4 cup flour
1 pound ground turkey breast
2 tablespoons salt-free Cajun spice blend (see recipe below), divided
1/4 teaspoon cayenne, or more if needed

¼ teaspoon bottled liquid smoke (available in most supermarkets)

3 tablespoons minced garlic, divided

2 tablespoons canola oil, divided

4 ribs celery, thinly sliced

2 large onions, diced

2 red bell peppers, diced

2 green bell peppers, diced

8 cups fat-free chicken broth

8 ounces okra, tops trimmed and cut into 1-inch pieces

1 bay leaf

1 pound medium shrimp (thawed if frozen), peeled and deveined

salt and pepper, to taste

Preheat oven to 400°F. Spread flour on a baking sheet and toast in oven for 45 to 60 minutes or until nut brown, stirring occasionally. Sift into a bowl and set aside.

Meanwhile, make turkey "andouille" sausage. Thoroughly combine ground turkey, 1 tablespoon Cajun seasoning, cayenne, liquid smoke, and 1 tablespoon garlic. Form into small patties, about ½ tablespoon each. Heat 1 tablespoon oil in a large, heavy skillet or Dutch oven. Brown sausage patties on both sides. Remove and set aside.

Add remaining oil to pan and heat. Cook celery, onions, peppers, and remaining garlic until soft, about 10 minutes. Sprinkle flour over vegetables a little at a time, stirring between additions. Cook 2 minutes more. Slowly pour in broth while stirring. Add okra, bay leaf, and remaining Cajun seasoning. Stir in sausage. Bring to a boil, reduce heat, and simmer for 20 minutes. Skim foam from top of stew as it rises. Add shrimp and cook just long enough so that shrimp become opaque, about 5 to 10 minutes. Season to taste with pepper, and salt if sodium is not an issue.

Serve with cooked white or brown rice.

Per serving: 168 calories, 4g fat (17.2% calories from fat), 25g protein, 14g carbohydrate, 2g dietary fiber, 79mg cholesterol, 480mg sodium.

Salt-Free Cajun Spice Blend

Yield: ⅔ cup

8 teaspoons paprika

4 teaspoons granulated garlic

4 teaspoons granulated onion

4 teaspoons ground black pepper

2 teaspoons ground white pepper

1 to 2 teaspoons cayenne

2 teaspoons dried oregano, rubbed

2 teaspoons dried basil, rubbed

2 teaspoons dried thyme, rubbed

¼ teaspoon celery seed

Combine all ingredients well and place in airtight container.

Low-Fat Sweet Potato Pie with Pecan Crust

There are several ingredients that drive up the calorie count of a pie: butter (and/or shortening) in the crust, lots of eggs, maybe cream, and more butter. This recipe sidesteps all those calorie traps with a few clever substitutes like orange juice (to hold the crust together) and evaporated skim milk.

Serves 8

Have on hand:
food processor
9-inch pie plate
medium bowl

FOR CRUST

- ¼ cup pecans, chopped
- 1½ cups graham cracker crumbs
- ¼ cup Grape-Nuts cereal
- 3 tablespoons orange juice

FOR FILLING

- 2 cups mashed sweet potatoes
- ½ cup evaporated skim milk
- 1 egg, lightly beaten
- 1 egg white, lightly beaten
- ½ cup maple syrup
- ½ teaspoon ground cinnamon
- ¼ teaspoon ground nutmeg

Preheat oven to 350°F.

Finely chop the pecans in a food processor. Add graham cracker crumbs and Grape-Nuts. With machine running, slowly add orange juice until mixture begins to come together (add 1 additional tablespoon orange juice if needed).

Press crumbs evenly into a 9-inch pie plate. Bake in preheated oven for 12 to 16 minutes, or until dry. Set aside to cool.

Increase oven temperature to 400°F. Stir together pie-filling ingredients in a medium bowl until well combined. Pour into crust, and bake in preheated oven for 10 minutes. Reduce temperature to 350°F and continue baking for 50 to 60 minutes or until a knife inserted 1 inch from the center comes away clean. Cool for 2 hours before slicing.

Per serving: *244 calories, 5 g fat (17% calories from fat), 5 g protein, 46 g carbohydrate, 2 g dietary fiber, 24 mg cholesterol, 202 mg sodium.*

Perfect Peach Cobbler

Peach pie is one of my absolute favorites. I don't have the real thing too often anymore, but I'm happy with this substitute: super delicious and a lot less damaging to the waistline.

Serves 8

Have on hand:
2-quart baking dish
canola oil cooking spray
medium mixing bowl
large saucepan
wire cooling rack

1 cup HeartSmart Bisquick baking mix
2 tablespoons sugar
1/2 teaspoon ground cinnamon
1/4 teaspoon ground ginger
1/2 cup evaporated skim milk
5 cups fresh or frozen and thawed peach slices
2 tablespoons finely chopped crystallized ginger
1/2 cup packed brown sugar
1 tablespoon cornstarch
1/4 cup water

Preheat oven to 400°F. Lightly spray a shallow 2-quart baking dish with canola oil spray, and set aside.

In a medium bowl, stir together baking mix, sugar, cinnamon, ground ginger, and milk until just combined. Set aside. In a large saucepan, combine peaches, crystallized ginger, and brown sugar. Stir cornstarch into water until dissolved, then add to the pan. Cook over medium heat until thickened and bubbly.

Transfer peaches to prepared baking dish and drop spoonfuls of sweet biscuit dough over fruit. Bake for 20 to 25 minutes or until topping is cooked through. Cool cobbler on a wire cooling rack for 1 hour before serving. If desired, serve with a dollop of light whipped topping or a small scoop of vanilla low-fat frozen yogurt.

Per serving: *289 calories, 1 g fat (3.9% calories from fat), 3 g protein, 69 g carbohydrate, 3 g dietary fiber, 1 mg cholesterol, 163 mg sodium.*

CHAPTER TWO

A Musician's Life—Fast Times, Fast Food

In Louisiana there's only one thing they love as much as food, and that's music. For me, music was like food of a different kind—food for the soul. I fell in love with it at an early age. My older brother played drums and held band practice in our garage, and that's where I developed a thing for the bass. I tried playing drums like my brother. I tried playing guitar, and I played saxophone and keyboards for a while, but the bass really spoke to me. At the time I was listening to all the early Motown stuff, James Brown, Sam & Dave, Hank Williams, Jimi Hendrix, Led Zeppelin, and the Beatles. I mean, Paul McCartney! He's an amazing bass player, one of the legends of our time. I was open to all kinds of music as long as it was good.

But my real inspiration in those days was a neighborhood guy named Sammy Thorton who played bass with a local band called Big Bo Melvin & the Nighthawks ("cuz you got to do all your hawking at night"). The Nighthawks would rehearse on Sammy's front porch, and even though I was only about thirteen years old he let me hang with them and schooled me in the electric bass. It was as great an introduction to the instrument as you could ever hope for.

Once I got a handle on the bass, I started playing whenever and wherever I could. At weddings. At church. Anywhere they would let me. At the age of fifteen I started sneaking into bars and playing with the bands. I had to hide behind my amp so that I wouldn't get thrown out for being (way) below drinking age. But alcohol wasn't the only reason I probably shouldn't have been in there. These bars were wild! Some of them were located across the railroad tracks in the deep hood, and there would be gunshots, knifings, and all kinds of dangerous stuff going on. It always seemed like there'd be a guy in there, the "undertaker," who'd brought his ambulance because he knew something was going to go down, whether it be a shooting, a stabbing, or someone breaking off a bottle neck and using it as a weapon. Whatever, this guy was there, ready to pick up the pieces.

Everyone was very passionate about drinking, dancing, women, and song, so these nights could get pretty out of control. And it was a fairly classic scenario in the South: the eagle flies on Friday (meaning, you get paid and use the cash to carry on and let off steam) then by the time Monday rolls around, stormy Monday, you're broke again and singing the blues. T-Bone Walker wrote a song called "Stormy Monday" about it, and it's been recorded by many artists, including Eric Clapton and B. B. King.

Yeah, those bars were pretty raucous, but they also had great food. I may not have been drinking at that age, but I was eating. I remember a few hot sausage sandwiches, with mustard, on a white bread bun that were out of this world. Food and music, I was just beginning to learn, go together pretty well.

When I enrolled in Southern University at Baton Rouge, with a double major in music and psychology, I kept right on performing. I was still working out and hanging out with athletes, but I wasn't playing football or running track anymore. Music had mostly overtaken my life. Gradually I stopped exercising and, not surprisingly, started gaining weight. I was no longer a big athlete; just on my way to becoming a big man. For a long time I'd been called Fat Cat, because I was big and I had, you know, that cool, cocky, fat-cat demeanor. But by the time I graduated from college, I was starting to become a fat cat in the more literal sense of the word.

I've got to say, though, that I didn't really notice or care too much at the time. I was in the zone, man, thinking only about what gigs I could get. I think this is something a lot of people who've gone from normal weight to overweight experience. You just get busy with life and the things you are passionate about, whether it's your work or your family or both, and you don't pay attention to what's happening to your body. You eat with assumed impunity and sit on your butt without worrying about how big that butt is getting. Then one day you wake up and realize that, hey, these pants don't fit so well, or you go to the doctor's and cringe when you see the numbers on the scale. Why the big surprise? You've been stuffing your face. But, then again, it's really easy to ignore what's happening or, if you're aware of it, to kid yourself. "It's not so bad." You look in the mirror, stand up straight so your stomach tucks in, and go out and get on with your life.

Then there's the age part of it. Maybe when you were young you could eat like a maniac and not gain an ounce. But as you get into your twenties and start working a job, maybe one where you sit at a desk, or one like mine where going out to eat after work is part of the ritual, the pounds start creeping on. Your metabolism, the number of calories you burn per day, changes as you get older too. So then there's this huge disconnect. *I've always eaten a burger and fries for lunch and had ice cream after dinner. You going to tell me I can't do that anymore?* It takes a while for your mind to catch up with what's happening to your body—and even longer to realize that you've got to change your ways.

Once my musical career began to take off, weight was the last thing I was thinking about. I was living the life and loving it. At eighteen, when I was just starting college, I got my first big break when I joined John Fred & His Playboy Band. The group was popular in the South and had scored a number one national hit in 1964 with the song "Judy in Disguise (with Glasses)," a parody of the Beatles' "Lucy in the Sky with Diamonds." A few years later, at age twenty, I got a taste of what it was like to go on tour when Mahavishnu Orchestra drummer Billy Cobham hired me. Soon after, I hooked up with the jazz fusion violinist Jean-Luc Ponty, then in the early eighties I joined the band Journey.

During this time I was doing a lot of in-studio recording gigs (called session work, in music biz lingo). I played with Carlos Santana and Jerry Garcia of the Grateful Dead and collaborated with producer Narada Michael Walden on hits like Whitney Houston and Aretha Franklin's "Who's Zoomin' Who?" as well as the singers' separate hits "Freeway of Love" (Franklin) and "I Wanna Dance with Somebody (Who Loves Me)" (Houston). In the short span of a few years, I had gone from down-home kid playing high school football to fast-lane adult performing in huge, sold-out arenas of twenty-five thousand screaming fans.

I was getting to work with pretty amazing people too. People always ask me, "Who was the best artist you've ever worked with?" "Who was the nicest?" "Who was the meanest?" I always disappoint, because it's so hard to narrow it down. I have had the good fortune to work with so many great artists. What I can say for sure is that working with Mariah Carey was a dream; Whitney Houston was a dream; Aretha Franklin was a dream. I loved working with Bruce Springsteen, Madonna, and Justin Timberlake—they are all just madly talented. Some former *Idol* contestants, too, rank right up there as great people to work with. Katharine McPhee and Elliot Yamin are awesome. I thought of them immediately when I was putting together my album *Randy Jackson's Music Club, Volume 1.*

Anyhow, when I got to the point where my career was really on fire, I suddenly found myself riding in private jets, receiving the attention of ladies more beautiful than I'd ever imagined, and partying like crazy. Yes, I partied like everyone else. At one time I was a pretty good drinker. I could hold my liquor pretty well. Yeah, I drank that oil. But I eventually let go of that and the other vices that tend to go hand in hand with rock and roll. I'm happy to say that my partying never got too out of control. I probably would have been thinner (though obviously not healthier) if it did! It's no secret that a lot of rock-and-roll guys do drugs, and it's one reason why they stay so skinny. They feed their addictive proclivities with drugs and alcohol, not food. For me it was more of the opposite. I ate partly out of a natural inclination toward excess, partly out of boredom, and partly because—like Mount Everest, baby—that food was *there*.

Real-Life Alert
In the Midnight Hours: How Bad Is Late-Night Eating?

When you're a musician, there are no two ways about it: you're going to eat late at night. Most musicians live a pretty upside-down life because they might get off work anywhere between 10:00 p.m. and what Frank Sinatra called the "wee small hours of the morning." It's almost like being a night-shift worker.

I couldn't do anything about eating late when I was still a full-time musician, but now I live a more normal nine-to-five (okay, nine-to-seven) kind of life. On *Idol* days I split my time between my office/studio and the set where we shoot the show. But even then I'm usually done in the early evening. One thing that hasn't changed much since my younger years is that I still eat away from home a lot. When you're in the music business, it's the nature of the beast: Everybody is always wanting to do dinner meetings, or some celebrity is launching a restaurant and my wife and I are invited to the opening. Then there are movie premieres and concerts—you've got to go to these things to stay on top of who's hot (and because, well, they're fun). My life might not be called normal in small-town America, but it's a lot quieter than it was when I was burning the candle at both ends.

Still, I don't eat dinner by 6:00 p.m., and that seems to go against common weight-loss advice. I've always wondered if it's really as important as they say, not to eat past that particular witching hour. Or is that just more diet hype? I asked Erin Naimi, and here's what she had to say.

"Your metabolism does get a little slower at night, but it doesn't shut down," explains Erin. "That's not the problem with eating after 6:00 p.m. The reason night eating is considered problematic is because it's usually linked to sitting in front of the TV and snacking mindlessly." A lot of people who are bored or lonely at night use food to get a sense of stimulation or nurturing.

So in that sense, night eating isn't healthy. But Erin doesn't see not eating dinner until seven, eight, or even ten o'clock as a problem as long as it's not a matter of endless grazing throughout the night. "I think it's better to eat dinner than to go without, because eventually you will get very hungry and that's going to put you at risk for bingeing later on," she says.

Okay, but what if it's two o'clock in the morning and you're coming home hungry from a club or a party?

If you have something like a piece of string cheese or a piece of fruit, it's not really a problem. "But usually when people are eating at two in the morning, they're sitting in a café having a tuna melt and fries, and that of course can be a problem if you're trying to lose weight," says Erin. It can be a matter of perception, though. Keep in mind that a piece of string cheese or a piece of fruit will probably satisfy you. Just because it's 2:00 a.m. doesn't mean that you should throw out the choices you'd make by the light of day.

During those rock-and-roll years, a lot of the time I wasn't even conscious of how much I was eating. Late at night I'd come off a gig and go back to my hotel room, where it would be quiet and I'd have nothing to do. I'd be wired and unable to go to bed, in a town where I knew no one. So what was I going to do? God knows I wasn't going to work out. I'd start looking at the room service menu, and then next thing I know I'd be on the phone ordering way too many things. By the time the food arrived, I'd be so hungry that I'd eat and eat until I was stuffed. Remember, I grew up in a family where you ate as much as possible. You didn't want to go disrespecting the cook by not finishing your food. My habit was to finish what was on my plate, hungry or not.

That's what often went on when I was alone, though I spent many nights socializing after a gig. That was a food trap too. When you're on the road with a band, eating is a communal part of the experience. And you're always having food thrown at you. It starts at the sound check, during the day before a performance, when you make sure the audio system is working right. The venue you're playing at has the deli tray out for you, and when you come back for the gig there's even more food. After the show, friends come backstage, and everybody hangs out and eats (and drinks). You're chatting and mingling, not paying much attention to what you're eating, and before you know it, you've had two sandwiches and double desserts.

It's easy to do because there's always a big smorgasbord backstage. There are all kinds of sandwiches—the type that have about 2,500 calories stuffed into a little package—plus chips, cheeses, cookies, cakes, candy, beer, wine. They always have what you like because the band's management puts your requests on something called a venue rider. If we wanted M&M's and fried chicken at every arena we played, it was on the rider.

It's not all that different from the buffets you find at hotels when you're on vacation. In those days I thought buffets were great, but now I see them as crazy, deadly! Buffets are the enemy. Too much of anything is terrible for you, and those buffets are just so tempting. Now I avoid them like them like I avoid a rabid dawg.

Even the less fancy gigs can evolve into eating extravaganzas. You have just finished playing for three or four hours and, wow, you're tired and hungry. Man, let's go eat. That's when you hang out with the guys, shoot the shit, talk about the night. I'd often use going out after playing as a time to talk to the older guys, get some advice, and become chummy with them so that maybe they'd hire me for their next gig. In the South and Midwest that would generally mean that we'd head over to a waffle house. You can always find a good waffle house in the South and Midwest. I'd have chicken and waffles or hash browns smothered and covered: gravy, syrup, butter, cheese—whatever you wanted or could possibly think of—piled on top!

The other day in LA, I was out having breakfast and saw a woman gingerly putting a little syrup on her pancakes. That's not how Southerners eat them. In the South, those pancakes would be swimming in syrup. Not only that, they'd have butter oozing all over them. Dude, every meal is a possible heart attack but, oh my God, does it taste good!

Throughout my career as a musician on tour (which isn't over—I still go out when the spirit moves me and the artist is as amazing as Mariah Carey), I played all around the world and throughout the country. The Meadowlands in New Jersey. The Cow Palace in San Francisco. We hit all kinds of venues, big and small.

If I had to pick a favorite place to play, I would say Dallas and New Orleans. Texans seem to really enjoy it when musical acts come to their town. I'm not sure what it is about them—maybe they're not as jaded as people in some of the bigger cities—but Texans are great to perform for. Then again, I love playing Soldier Field in Chicago, Madison Square Garden in New York, and the Gibson Amphitheatre in LA. When you love playing, they're all good, and you don't care about the money. Only business guys think about that. Not true artists.

I'm sure the Dave Matthews Band loves playing anywhere they can. The Grateful Dead never turned up their noses and said, "We're not going to play in this ratty park." When you love playing, you love playing.

If playing some of those fancier arenas and theaters sounds glamorous, well it is—up to a point. A lot about touring with a big artist is decidedly unglamorous. When you're on the road for weeks and months at a time, there are many, many hours spent on a cramped bus with not much to do. And the food can be dismal. A lot of times you eat just for convenience or because you're bored. So you can imagine that when occasional opportunities to travel on a private jet came up, I was thrilled. Instead of eating some junk you picked up when the bus stopped at a 7-Eleven, you would sit in the lap of luxury with catered meals and whatever your heart desires. It's like what I imagine Roman banquets were like: Caesar's eating the whole leg of the biggest turkey on the planet, stuffing himself until he finally passes out. A feast.

But, again, that was only once in a while. Most of the time when you're touring with a band, you're stuck on that big confining bus, traveling from town to town. As I mentioned earlier, the bus is usually stocked with food (not a lot of it healthy), but a lot of fast-food eating goes on too. Maybe you know what I'm talking about. You're traveling with friends or family, and the choices on the road are pretty limited. You find yourself stopping at a fast-food hub and loading up on burgers, fries, and shakes, not only to ease the tedium of the trip, but because you never know what other restaurants lie down the highway. This might be your last chance for a while!

What's the Damage?
A Little Fast-Food Reality Check

I'm glad that a lot of fast-food restaurants have healthier choices now, but back in my touring days the options were slim—and guaranteed to make you fat. Of course you can still get all those heart-attack-on-a-bun meals today, but compare them with smarter options and you'll see that you don't have to pay such a high price for low-budget food.

The Killer Fast-Food Option	The Healthier Fast-Food Option
Bean and cheese burrito with steak OR Half order chips and guacamole + Medium cola	Two soft chicken tacos Mexican rice + Water
1,740 calories	570 calories
Fried chicken breast and drumstick OR Mashed potatoes with gravy Cole slaw Pecan pie + Medium Mountain Dew	Roast chicken sandwich Corn on the cob Baked beans + Medium Diet Coke
1,140 calories	610 calories

The Killer **Fast-Food Option**		**The Healthier** **Fast-Food Option**
Quarter-pound hamburger	OR	Hamburger
Medium fries		Salad with ranch dressing
+ Medium chocolate shake		+ Child's-size Sprite (12 oz)
1,350 calories		660 calories
Biscuit with sausage, egg, and cheese	OR	Scrambled eggs Low-fat muffin
Hash browns		+ Orange juice
+ Coffee		540 calories
710 calories		

Source: http://www.washingtonpost.com/wp-srv/flash/health/calorie counter/counter.htm

This is the kind of thing everyone faces, but when you're on tour with a band, you face it to the nth degree. Those fast-food places just keep coming at you, and far be it from me to refuse what they had to offer. Trust me, I never ordered the grilled chicken sandwich or the salad (of course, in those days not a lot of places even offered grilled chicken sandwiches and salads). Truck stops had some pretty enjoyable food too, especially the chili and corn bread.

One thing I can say for sure about those days is that I had blast. I had a blast every time I went out on a tour, every gig I played. I felt so fortunate to be earning a living in music because I was so passionate about it—and I still am. What an opportunity. I mean, wait a minute: We're out on tour. There are a bunch of chicks following us around. We're drinking. We're eating everything in sight. We're on stage and playing and people love us. And I'm getting paid for it. Thank you, God! Let me do this for the rest of my life!

What I'm saying is that you couldn't tell me that anything was wrong with all that. You couldn't tell me that having a steak dripping with butter, a baked potato stuffed with everything under the sun, and salad hidden under a chunk of blue cheese was bad. Everything was good.

Until, of course, it wasn't.

Chicken Étouffée

This Cajun dish is often made with crawfish—and a whole mess o' butter. Here, you use a tiny bit of butter, just enough to add flavor, but not enough to drive up your cholesterol count.

Serves 4

Have on hand:
large nonstick skillet

> **6 tablespoons flour**
> **2 teaspoons salt-free Cajun spice blend (see recipe on page 16)**
> **1 teaspoon poultry seasoning**
> **1½ pounds boneless skinless chicken breasts, cut into 1-inch pieces**

1 teaspoon canola oil
2 teaspoons unsalted butter
1½ cups finely chopped onion
1 cup finely chopped green bell pepper
¾ cup finely chopped celery
2 cups fat-free chicken broth
salt and pepper, to taste

Toast flour in a large nonstick skillet over medium-high heat. Watch flour carefully so that it doesn't burn. Frequently shake pan and stir until flour turns a dark nut color, about 10 to 15 minutes. Sift flour into a bowl; set aside.

Combine Cajun and poultry seasoning, and toss with chicken until evenly coated. Add oil and butter to a large skillet over medium-high heat. When butter has melted, add chicken and brown on all sides. Transfer to a plate and set aside.

Add vegetables to the pan and sweat until softened, about 6 to 8 minutes. Sprinkle flour over vegetables a little at a time, stirring between additions. Once flour has been added, slowly stir in broth until well combined. Return chicken to the pan and bring mixture to a boil. Reduce heat to a simmer and cook for 10 to 15 minutes, or until chicken is cooked through. If sauce becomes too thick, add water 1 tablespoon at a time to loosen. Season to taste with pepper, and salt if sodium is not an issue.

Serve hot over cooked white or brown rice.

Per serving: *303 calories, 5 g fat (15.9% calories from fat), 47 g protein, 18 g carbohydrate, 3 g dietary fiber, 104 mg cholesterol, 383 mg sodium.*

Banana Pudding Pie

I never thought I'd find a substitute for banana cream pie, one of my all-time favorites. But this pared-down version is incredibly creamy—though it doesn't have a drop of cream. A worthy alternative to the real thing.

Serves 8

Have on hand:
food processor
9-inch glass pie plate
small mixing bowl
whisk
electric mixer

FOR CRUST

2 cups reduced-fat Nilla wafer crumbs (about 55 cookies)
¼ cup chopped walnuts
¼ cup orange juice

FOR FILLING

1 package sugar-free vanilla pudding and pie filling (6-serving size)
2½ cups evaporated skim milk
½ teaspoon rum or vanilla extract
3 bananas, sliced ¼-inch thick

FOR OPTIONAL MERINGUE TOPPING
  ½ cup pasteurized egg whites
  ½ teaspoon rum or vanilla extract
  ¼ teaspoon cream of tartar
  4 tablespoons powdered sugar

Preheat oven to 350°F.

Place Nilla wafer crumbs and walnuts in a food processor and pulse until you have a fine crumb. With the motor running, add orange juice 1 tablespoon at a time until the crumbs are moist and will hold together (add an additional tablespoon of orange juice if necessary). Evenly press crumbs into the bottom and up the sides of a 9-inch pie plate. Bake in preheated oven for 15 to 20 minutes or until crust is dry and hard. Set aside to cool.

In a small mixing bowl, whisk together pudding mix, evaporated milk, and rum extract for 2 minutes, until smooth. Line bottom and sides of pie crust with banana slices and spread with half of the pudding. Top with remaining banana slices and spread with remaining pudding. Let set in refrigerator 1 hour before slicing.

Optional meringue topping: Beat together egg whites, rum extract, and cream of tartar with an electric mixer until soft peaks form. Add sugar and beat to stiff, but not dry, peaks. Spread meringue over chilled pie, making sure that the meringue seals to the crust. Bake in preheated oven for 15 to 20 minutes or until golden brown.

Per serving: 284 calories, 5 g fat (14.1% calories from fat), 10 g protein, 53 g carbohydrate, 1 g dietary fiber, 3 mg cholesterol, 448 mg sodium.

CHAPTER THREE

Diary of a Serial Dieter

I f you watched the first two seasons of *American Idol*, you know that I looked almost like a different guy back then. I barely recognize myself when I look at the old shows. Naturally, when I showed up for Season 3 considerably leaner, everyone was pretty surprised. Simon and Paula knew that I was going to have surgery, and they were very supportive, as was everyone else on the show. And they loved seeing me looking so much healthier. "Dude, you are the bomb!" Well, at least that's how I felt.

The thing is, although my transformation might have seemed abrupt to viewers, I had been trying to lose weight for a long time. I'm not a diet expert—but I *am* an expert on dieting. My experience in the area is vast. I have tried them all, but by the time I was a regular on *Idol* those diets were failing me. Or I was failing them. Whichever. It all amounts to the same thing in the end: diets absolutely do not work.

Now, I'm not talking about moderating your calories, resizing your portions, making healthier choices, and eating less of your favorite (i.e., fattening) foods. That's not a diet; that's adopting a new and healthier lifestyle, which I encourage you to do. What I mean by "diet" is a program that has you slashing calories drastically so that you drop a lot of pounds right away, look in the mirror, and say, "Damn, I look fine," then go back to eating the way you did before. Next thing you know, you're fat again. Oops. Then there are the diets that require so much work—counting protein grams; fixing special, hard-to-find foods; measuring out meager ounces—that you end up tossing out the book. Who's got the time for all that?

When I read that researchers at UCLA found that 41 percent of dieters gained back more weight then they lost in the first place, it didn't surprise me because I've experienced it firsthand. When you say you're *on* a diet, that means you can fall *off* the diet. I can't tell you how many diets I've been on. And off. Zone. Weight Watchers. Scarsdale. Atkins. (And I'm not alone. The American Society for Metabolic and Bariatric Surgery found that people who have weight-loss surgery try an average of twenty-four diet and exercise programs before going under the knife.) I started dieting when I was in my twenties. Although I put my head in the sand for a long time, I finally had to face the fact that all that "social eating" backstage, on-the-road fast food, and general Southern-boy overindulgence had made my body bigger than ever. After one of my first tours with Journey, I decided to try a liquid fast. I had no idea what I was in for.

Going on a liquid fast is not as hard as it sounds. I'm not

advocating it—noooo no no. I'm just saying that when you cut out all food, or almost all food (some fasts let you have a meal a day), it actually becomes kind of easy after a while. But that's not necessarily a good thing. In fact, those long-term fasts can be very deceptive.

The fast I tried was OPTIFAST, which was very popular back then. I drank only shakes for about five months. After the first couple of weeks, your appetite actually starts to diminish so, while it sounds like it's really hard to survive only on liquids, it gets easier as you go along. By the time I went off the diet, I was down to 150 pounds. Now, I'm five foot eleven so that is skinny. At first I was kind of excited. Wow, I'm a skinny guy! But then I realized something: I am not a skinny guy. I mean psychologically. That's just not me. I didn't feel like myself.

I didn't really look like myself either. I'd look in the mirror and say to myself, "Who the hell is that?" Other people didn't quite get it either. Sure, some would say, "You look great," but those who really knew me would say things like, "You look emaciated," "You look weird," or "My God, your head is ginormous!" And it was. Being so thin made my head look huge. Like I was wearing a bucket. When you have lived most of your life as a heavy person, it's hard to live life as a skinny person, and that's what I ran up against. I had gone too far.

That's probably part of the reason that I ended up gaining the weight back in about six months. The rest of the reason? Who can live on shakes for his entire life? I went right back to eating like I always had. That's what I knew. I hadn't tried out any healthier habits during that fast or given myself time to get used to lower calorie foods. I didn't practice listening to my body's signals so that I'd know when I was truly hungry or full. It was kind of an either-or situation. I was either fasting or overeating, no in-between.

Over the years, I alternated dieting with overeating. I never went back to the OPTIFAST, but I tried other things, including weight-loss drugs and B_{12} shots in the butt. The drugs I tried were the kind that speed you up. You don't want to eat, and you have all this extra energy, which sounds great until you crash and burn. Believe me, it's not worth the scary heart palpitations.

I've also done juice fasts for about ten days. They aren't for everybody (and you've got to check in with your doctor about fasting if you're ever inclined to try one), but I do see some merit in them. What happens is that you lose mostly water weight, but those ten or twelve pounds get your attention. Your energy lifts, and some of your cravings stop, so that when the ten days are over you've gotten kind of a jump start. You feel good and are ready to start living a healthier life. It's somewhat like what a gastric bypass does for you (I'll tell you more about that later), though of course on a much smaller scale. (Not everyone thinks fasting is so great; see page 104 for a dietitian's take on fasts.)

The tricky thing with a juice fast is that you can't just come off of it and think that your work is done. That's the problem with most diets. Being on a diet is kind of like being in prison: it's all about deprivation. When you've served your time and get out of prison, *you're not supposed to go back to your old tricks.*

Likewise, when you go off a diet, you're not supposed to go back to eating three-inch-thick roast beef sandwiches and pasta drowned in cream sauce. The trouble is that most people do go right back to eating in the same criminally unhealthy fashion. I did it a hundred times. On a diet, off a diet—and eating poorly again.

Real-Life Alert
Confronting the Coffeehouse Pastry Case

If you live in one of the rare places on earth that doesn't have a Starbucks, you probably have some kind of equivalent. We have a gajillion Starbucks and about six other chains around town, and that's not including all the independent places. There seem to be two coffeehouses on every corner now. I often find myself in one of them, either with my kids or for an informal meeting with someone, and each time I walk in it tests my resolve. Because, of course, there under the little spotlights and shiny glass are plates full of muffins, cookies, cakes, and croissants, beckoning with a come-hither stare.

"But were you even thinking about getting a cookie or muffin before you went in there? Did you just want some tea or did you want a chocolate croissant?" asks Erin. Uh, good point. I wasn't going in for a pastry, and I try to keep that in mind whenever those seductive little sweets try to break my determination to eat healthfully. In order to be less impulsive and more deliberate, I take a step back and recall my original intention. I take a deep breath and walk around the place for minute. By the time I circle back, the craving usually subsides. If the pastries have really got me going and all of a sudden I'm genuinely hungry, I try to look past them to the sandwiches, yogurt, or the little fruit or vegetable platters that a lot of places sell. Nine times out of ten there's going to be something fairly healthy in that coffeehouse, but it's hard to see it when your eyes are blinded by the light of a heavily frosted cinnamon bun.

The expression "your eyes are bigger than your stomach" is absolutely true. Dude, we all live in an ocular fantasy world! The fancy clothes, the racy car, the big houses—in our eyes they all look amazing. In reality, of course, they're not always so.

Most times I find that the pause and deep breath I take helps me pass on the pastries. If I can't forget about them, then I go ahead and have one and I don't beat myself up about it. I know it's not going to kill me because I'm not having those muffins and croissants every day. But before I reapproach the counter, I also ask myself this: are those pastries really that good? A lot of times those coffeehouse baked goods really aren't that great. They're either stale and dry or just not made with high-quality ingredients. It's as though they were an afterthought. I try to remember that, because when I treat myself, I want it to be worth it.

All my dieting experience has taught me a lot, and most especially this: forget diets. And the ones that promise you a new body in ten days are the worst offenders. Instead, change your eating habits and get off the couch and start moving to burn some calories. But do it in a way that you're going to be able to maintain, that's realistic for you. And stop checking the calendar.

If you're in a hurry, you're going to make all the mistakes that lead to failure. How many times have you said to yourself, "Oh my God, I've got to lose thirty pounds before our anniversary party"? How about, "I've got to get my high school body back before I go to my reunion." Or, "I'm not going to get into a bathing suit this summer unless I'm fifty pounds lighter." I love all those diet come-ons for women that start showing up around May: "Get bikini beach body ready." "Want to look hot on the beach?" Why are you doing it for the beach? You should be losing weight for a healthier life, not to look hot for the few hours you're going to be hanging out on the sand. Or to pick up guys or girls.

Or for the few hours that you'll be wearing a wedding dress. I recently read about a study at Cornell University that found that 70 percent of women were trying to lose weight for their wedding day. A lot of them were taking diet pills, fasting, and skipping meals just to get into that gown (some of them had even bought a dress a size smaller as incentive). Hey, you know, everyone wants to look good walking down the aisle; there's nothing wrong with that. What I'm saying is that when you try to lose weight for an event without looking at the bigger picture—and by that I mean, is losing weight quick going to help you keep it off for life?—you are likely to gain the weight back. How many people have lost weight for their wedding only to put half the pounds back on before the honeymoon is over? A few months later they've gained twice the weight. Quick-fix diets always come back to haunt you.

A Glass of Water, a Bowl of Soup, a Stick of Gum: Can You Deceive Your Stomach?

Sometimes I feel hungry when I don't want to be. Maybe I just ate, so I know that what I'm experiencing isn't true physical hunger (more on this in chapter 5), or maybe I'm somewhere where there are no healthy choices to be found. So I do either one of two things: have a glass of water or chew gum.

Does it work? Somewhat. Take the water. I do try to get in the recommended eight glasses of water a day. The human body is 70 percent water, so it's important to keep replenishing the supply. Besides, I can feel the difference if I let myself get dehydrated. Drinking a lot of water seems to help keep me in balance. And it does relieve my hunger a little. It doesn't make me so full that I'm going to forget about lunch, but it helps tide me over when I need it.

What works even better, but along the same lines, is soup. The liquid in it seems to fill me up more than comparably sized amounts of food. I often start a meal with something like asparagus or broccoli soup (provided they're not made with cream—that would defeat the purpose), and it seems to help me eat less of the rest of my meal. Back in the old days when I'd go on diets, some of them would have you eat some god-awful cabbage broth or vegetable bouillon made from a salty cube. But the soups I eat today are different. They're made with fresh herbs or ginger, and they don't feel "diet-y." A lot of restaurants have great soups now, and even some big supermarkets have good choices at their soup and salad bars.

Gum is another appetite suppressant that I sometimes use to keep from eating. It has its limitations though. In the same way artificial sweeteners can trick your body into thinking it's getting food (see page 125 for more on artificial sweeteners), gum kind of gets all your digestive juices flowing. Eventually it catches up with you and you have to eat for real. But better to do so when you're in a situation where there are good choices available. If gum or water or a cup of chicken broth can help you ignore the vending machines at your office and make it through until dinnertime at your own (healthfully stocked) home, I'm all for it.

We all have an addiction to the "right now." We want everything right away; it's the human condition. I want to look better instantaneously. I want to put on that cute pair of sneakers and that dope outfit immediately, go out, and show off my new body—see if my life changes because of it. But the diets that give you the "right now"—meaning that they get you to lose a lot of water weight or maybe even cannibalize your muscle so that you quickly drop pounds—have a short shelf life. They're usually so crazy that you can't live that way for long. Inevitably you go back to your old style of eating and get fat all over again. Then do it again. And again. It's called yo-yo dieting.

Diets are temporary, and I don't like anything temporary. What I've found is that you're going to do much better if you forget about dieting and adopt some new, healthier eating habits that you can stick with—habits I'll share with you in chapters 5 and 6. These are practices that you need to adopt forever, not just for a few months. Of course, if you're used to measuring success in units of "right now," at first it's not going to seem like you're making much headway. That's something you've got to face up to and deal with. I see people all the time who have been at it for weeks, even months, and aren't happy with the way things are going. Girls wishing they were down to a size 6; guys hoping to slip into those pants with the thirty-two-inch waist. But you can't think like that. Weight that's going to stay lost comes in smaller increments than you're probably used to. Patience is essential.

Having patience is really difficult for a lot of people. I see it in the music business all the time. Some singers think they should be an overnight sensation; they don't realize that a lot of hard work goes into becoming a successful musician, much less a star. I suppose *American Idol* feeds this idea, in a way, because some of these kids *do* become overnight sensations. But that's a rarity. And, listen, you don't want to just become a one-hit wonder; in many cases, if you peak without toiling in the trenches for a while, you can end up as a "where is he now?" story in *People* magazine.

It's the same with the weight-loss quick fix. If you don't do the hard work, the success you have isn't going to stick. So be patient because the payoff—the end to yo-yoing body weight—is worth it. Now, sure, when, instead of going on a diet, you make moderate changes—like paring down your portion sizes a bit and eating at regular times so you don't get crazy hungry and eat with abandon—it takes longer to lose weight. On the other hand, you're going to be less likely to gain back the weight you lost because you can *get used to* moderate changes. Diets can feel like torture, and how long can anyone stick with that? If you go the slow-and-steady route, you don't have to turn your life around 360 degrees or try to be perfect—moves that inevitably set you up for failure. Again, I want to be real with you. It's not that it's easy, but it's not as hard as living on a salad and three hard-boiled eggs a day.

I guess the real problem I have with diets is that they're all about "don't." Maybe it's the rock and roller in me, but I hate the word *don't*. If you tell me I can't have something, it makes me want it that much more. Again, that's human nature. I see it in my kids. I can say to them, don't do this, don't do that, then kick back and look at my watch: a few minutes later they'll be doing exactly what I said not to do. Nobody likes to hear *don't*.

Hoppin' John Soup

Hoppin' John is a traditional Southern dish that's usually served for good luck on New Year's Day. This souped-up version is a lot less fatty (classic Hoppin' John is made with ham hocks or bacon) and is delicious served year round.

Serves 8

Have on hand:
soup pot

2 tablespoons extra-virgin olive oil

1 medium onion, finely chopped

1 medium bell pepper, finely chopped

2 stalks celery, finely chopped

2 cloves garlic, minced

1 pound ground turkey breast

2 tablespoons salt-free Cajun spice blend (see recipe on page 16)

1½ cups diced tomatoes (15-oz can)

4 cups fat-free chicken broth*

2 cups water, or more if needed

½ cup converted rice

1½ cups canned black-eyed peas (15-oz can), drained and rinsed

16-oz bag frozen collard greens (optional)

salt and pepper, to taste

*Note: To reduce sodium, replace some or all or the chicken broth with water. Each cup of canned fat-free chicken broth has more than 500 milligrams of sodium.

Heat oil in a soup pot over medium-high heat. Add vegetables and sauté until soft, about 5 minutes. Crumble in ground turkey and add Cajun seasoning. Stir frequently to break up turkey until cooked through. Add remaining ingredients except black-eyed peas and collard greens, if using, and bring to a boil.

Reduce heat and simmer for 15 minutes. Add black-eyed peas and, if using, collard greens, and simmer for another 15 minutes. Adjust seasoning with salt and pepper. Serve hot with plenty of Louisiana-style hot sauce.

Per serving: *285 calories, 5 g fat (14.8% calories from fat), 27 g protein, 35 g carbohydrate, 5 g dietary fiber, 32 mg cholesterol, 553 mg sodium.*

Double-Dipped Buttermilk Oven-Fried Chicken

I thought fried chicken was part of my past, never to cross my lips again. Turns out, I can live happily with the oven-fried version of the dish. It's a lot less greasy but no less delicious.

Serves 6

Have on hand:
large ziplock bag
large wire cooling rack
rimmed baking sheet
2 large shallow bowls
1 plate
vegetable oil cooking spray

6 chicken breast halves without skin (6 oz each)
1½ cups buttermilk
3 tablespoons Tabasco sauce
4 cloves garlic, minced
1 cup flour
1 tablespoon dried oregano
1 tablespoon dried thyme
1 teaspoon cayenne
1 teaspoon kosher salt (optional)
2½ cups crumbed cornflakes
2 eggs, lightly beaten

Remove skin from chicken and cut away any excess fat. Rinse chicken under cold water and pat dry with paper towels. Place chicken in a large ziplock bag; set aside.

Whisk together buttermilk, Tabasco, and garlic. Pour over chicken and turn to coat. Squeeze air from bag and seal. Marinate in refrigerator for at least 3 hours and up to 24 hours. Turn chicken occasionally.

Preheat oven to 350°F. Place a large wire cooling rack over a rimmed baking sheet; set aside.

Whisk together flour, oregano, thyme, and cayenne in a large shallow bowl (if sodium is not an issue, add the kosher salt to flour mixture). Place cornflakes in a separate shallow bowl.

Remove chicken from marinade, gently shake off excess buttermilk, and reserve ¼ cup marinade. Immediately dip in flour mixture; coat well (you will have leftover mixture). Set aside on a plate.

Discard flour from bowl, and whisk together beaten egg and ¼ cup of the buttermilk marinade. Dip flour-coated chicken into egg mixture and then into cornflake crumbs, coating each piece evenly (you will have leftover cornflakes). Set on wire rack and lightly spray each piece with cooking spray. Bake uncovered in preheated oven for 1 hour, until chicken is cooked through and crispy.

Per serving: 402 calories, 5 g fat (10.8% calories from fat), 36 g protein, 53 g carbohydrate, 2 g dietary fiber, 133 mg cholesterol, 584 mg sodium.

Quick-Cooking Creole-Style Sea Bass

This dish takes just 20 minutes to make. Even *I* could fit that into my schedule. If you want to make it even easier, serve it without the sauce (it's equally as good). Place a few limes wedges and steamed vegetables on the side and you're set.

Serves 4

Have on hand:
shallow bowl
large baking pan
canola oil cooking spray

2 teaspoons freshly ground black pepper
1 tablespoon Old Bay seafood seasoning
1/2 teaspoon dried thyme
1 tablespoon lemon juice
2 teaspoons Tabasco sauce, or more if needed
4 sea bass fillets (about 41/2 oz each)

Preheat the broiler (or grill). Position the rack 4 inches from the heat source.

Stir together the pepper, Old Bay, and thyme in shallow bowl. Sprinkle fish with lemon juice and Tabasco, then coat with the seasoning mixture. Set each fillet on a plate and let stand for 10 minutes.

Lightly spray a baking pan with cooking spray. Place the fillets in the pan. Broil (or grill) until the fish is opaque throughout when tested with a tip of a knife, about 8 to 10 minutes. Serve immediately with white or brown rice and steamed okra.

Per serving: *130 calories, 3 g fat (19% calories from fat), 24 g protein, 1 g carbohydrate, trace dietary fiber, 53 mg cholesterol, 149 mg sodium.*

CHAPTER FOUR

Diabetes, Then a Surgical Jump Start

Before that sunny Saturday when I landed in the emergency room and was diagnosed with diabetes, the state of my health was the last thing on my mind. I had given up touring as a musician and was working as a record company executive: first as vice president of artists & repertoire (A & R)/staff producer at Columbia Records, then as senior VP of A & R/staff producer at MCA. That's the kind of job—signing new acts and developing the careers of artists already on the label—that keeps you constantly busy. A fun kind of busy, but busy nonetheless. You're always trying to find the next big thing, which means you not only spend a lot of time listening to loads of demo CDs, traveling, and working in recording studios, you also have to be out there listening to artists in small clubs and bars. Sometimes that means hitting several places in one night. And, yes, it's the record biz, so you're schmoozing all the time. Being an A & R guy is a very social occupation, and you know what that means: lots of eating and drinking.

When you aren't being wined and dined by a band's managers, you're doing the wining and dining, trying to convince some great musical prospect to sign with your label. Later that night you'll sneak off to some little dive in the Valley, hoping to discover the next Mariah Carey, Avril Lavigne, or Green Day.

By the time I was working as an executive, I'd pretty much abandoned dieting. Diets had let me down so many times—why continue? At the same time I was living a much more sedentary life. I'd sit behind a desk all day, then if I wasn't going out to see a performance, I'd go home and collapse, exhausted. When I was playing music, I'd be out there every night, moving across the stage and working up a sweat. At least then I was burning off some of the calories I was taking in. Once I was in that desk job, though, it got harder and harder to make myself move. I've always loved tennis, so I'd play when I could, and I did make myself work out here and there, but it wasn't enough to keep me from getting bigger and bigger.

Still, I just put my weight problem out of my mind. Besides, I had a lot of other things to think about, including the possibility of joining a new television show about to be launched on the Fox network.

I had only heard a little bit about the British hit *Pop Idol* when my agent at the time, Jeff Frasco, called and said, "Hey, this show is really blowing up over there, and we're thinking about bringing it to America. Dude, if you're inclined, you should really try this. Would you want to be a judge?"

At first I thought it sounded a little corny. Music on TV had never been done all that well, and I was afraid the show would be cheesy. Jeff sent me a batch of tapes, and when I popped them in the VCR, I was mesmerized by the amateurs singing their hearts out, competing for the promise of a record deal. Wow. They blew me away. Those performers were heartbreaking, inspiring, and often downright hilarious.

I went down and met all the people at Fox and Fremantle (the company that produces the show). We just sat and chatted. I guess you could say it was an audition. Obviously it went well. They invited me on board and I said yes. I am always up for a challenge, so I thought I'd check it out. Still, no one had very high expectations for the American show, renamed *American Idol*, and in the back of my mind I was thinking, "I don't know if this thing is really going to work, but let's see."

One of the things that worked right away was the panel of judges. Simon, Paula, and I have good chemistry. I have known Paula for about twenty years. We worked on a Michael Bolton video together years ago, and she did some choreography and staging for Journey. I had never met Simon before, but I knew who he was because he was an A & R guy like myself, only in the UK. They tried out a bunch of different people for hosts, finally deciding on Ryan Secreast and Brian Dunkleman as cohosts. Then, of course, Ryan came back alone the following year. From the start, we just clicked.

So at the very least I thought being on *American Idol* might be a good time. I had no idea it was going to become a cultural phenomenon. Who did? And who can take credit for it? Success has a million mothers and fathers.

But before the juggernaut that is *American Idol* was to even appear on TV, there I was, working on a bunch of stuff and kicking with my family during my free time, when suddenly

I had the sword of Damocles—diabetes—hanging over my head. I can't say that I'd never been warned about the risk of getting diabetes: I'd been told by doctors that I had to watch what I ate and exercise more, and been reminded that I had a genetic predisposition to the disease. It ran in my family. But if you only go to the doctor every year and a half, or wait even longer between visits, which I often did, it's easy to forget that little talk your doc gave you in the office. Besides, at the time, with the tennis and my occasional workouts, I thought I was doing pretty well. At least I wasn't completely inactive. Of course I was also still spending most of my time sitting behind a desk, and still eating like it was going out of style. Business dinners at steak houses, take-out pasta lunches eaten in the studio, late-night doughnut runs after seeing a band—a couple friendly games of tennis and a few minutes on the treadmill couldn't make up for all the calories I was consuming. The writing was on the wall.

When I think about why I got diabetes, I chalk it up to my body basically saying, "Dude, you have been doing wrong for way too long!" It got tired of the way of I was treating it. Dr. Fran has a slightly more scientific explanation for what happened. According to Dr. Fran—Frances Kaufman, MD, who wrote the foreword to this book and whom I met through our shared commitment to diabetes prevention—type 2 diabetes occurs when the body's cells don't respond to insulin. (Type 1, a far less common form of diabetes, occurs when the body produces little or no insulin at all.) Insulin is a hormone produced by the pancreas that helps the body use glucose, a type of sugar. We get glucose, also called blood sugar, mostly from the carbohydrates we eat, and we need it to fuel virtually *everything*—every blink of the eye, every thought that crosses our minds.

When the cells first stop responding to insulin, the pancreas makes up for it by producing more of the hormone. But after a while the pancreas gets worn out from all that extra work and stops compensating so much. So now, not only is the insulin not working too well, the body's not producing much of it either. Without insulin to whisk glucose into the cells, it accumulates in the blood and blood sugar rises. That's most likely why my blood sugar number finally went off the charts.

It's also probably why I didn't notice anything for a long time. That whole process happens over the course of many years. You don't even know what's going on inside your own body, and your doctor might not even know, either. Then, suddenly, everything comes to a head. All those symptoms I had—having to pee all the time, extreme thirst, sleepiness, dizziness—were due to my body trying to get rid of all the sugar. The cells release fluid to flush out the sugar, says Dr. Fran, which makes you urinate, and then, as your body tries to replenish the fluids, makes you thirsty.

I wouldn't wish the hellish week that finally sent me to the emergency room on anyone, but I have to admit that I was lucky to catch the problem when I did. Some people end up in the ER not just with high blood sugar but with a stroke or heart attack. When I found that out, and learned more about the disease, I had to sit up and take notice. As I've mentioned, the complications of diabetes are pretty scary: heart disease, blindness, kidney failure, amputation. You get the picture. It's some serious stuff.

Both my parents had that "sugar," but you know how

parents are. They're protective; they don't tell you about all the bad stuff that's going down with them. And kids (no matter how old) often don't dig deeper when their parents are making like everything is okay. I knew diabetes was bad, but I guess I never really knew how bad.

Looking back, I had all the classic risk factors: Having family members with the disease. Being African American (we're 1.6 times more likely to get the disease than whites). Then there was, so to speak, the elephant in the room: my weight. I was too heavy, and that was one of the main reasons my system had gotten so whacked out. The experts are still trying to figure out why excess body fat can lead to diabetes, but they know for sure that in many cases it does. Some overweight people don't end up getting the disease, but I'm not that lucky. Man, I thought the dawg was invincible! Turns out, I'm not.

Stopping Diabetes Before It Starts

It's possible that you are on the path to diabetes and don't even know it. A lot of people are: about 54 million people in the U.S.* There's even a name for the object of this blissful ignorance—prediabetes—and the frightening thing is that it has no symptoms.

I wish I had known I had prediabetes, because if you

*Source: Centers for Disease Control and Prevention

do, you can cure it before it turns into full-blown diabetes. And what's really cool is that you don't have to take medication to get better. The research shows that as far as combating prediabetes is concerned, doing things like changing your diet and bumping up the amount of exercise you do is frequently more effective than drug therapy.

What's critical, though, is finding out if you have it. The reason it so often goes undiagnosed is that most people aren't motivated to get their blood sugar checked. (They feel fine, why should they?) But since the condition is symptomless, that's really the only way to get clued in. If you have some of the risk factors for diabetes listed below, don't wait. Get into your doctor's office soon, and ask for a blood glucose test. I can't stress that enough. Go to your doctor and let him or her figure out what's going on with you.

Diabetes Risk Factors
- A family history of the disease
- A body mass index (BMI) of 25 or higher (Body mass index refers to your weight as it relates to your height. To find yours go to: http://www.nhlbi.nih.gov/guidelines/obesity/bmi_tbl.htm.)
- You're older than forty-five
- High cholesterol, high triglyceride levels, or high blood pressure
- You are African American, Latino, Native American, Asian American, or a Pacific Islander
- You have had gestational diabetes or delivered a baby over nine pounds

Once I got the diagnosis of diabetes, my doctor started me immediately on oral medication to get my blood sugar down. I was able to go home from the hospital with the stipulation that I visit his office on Monday for a complete workup. And believe me, I obeyed! I knew I couldn't fool around anymore. Much as I hate going to the doctor, I went, and when I got there, he more or less read me the riot act. He told me I had to get my whole scene together. "This is a *serious* disease," he said. "It's nothing to play around with. You can manage diabetes, but in most cases there's no cure." Diabetes, he told me, can damage your kidneys, the blood vessels in your eyes, and the nerves in your feet. It tremendously increases your risk of developing cardiovascular disease. It is, in fact, the fifth-leading cause of death in the United States. When my doctor recommended that I see a nutritionist and start relearning how to eat, I knew I had to take his advice.

And so I got off on the right foot. I met with a nutritionist, and I did start eating right. Kind of. I cut way back on carbs, especially sugar (sugar, I was to discover, is in almost everything, including things you don't even think about, like ketchup and some kinds of bread). I started eating more salads, chicken instead of meat, and laying off all the gravy that I'd grown up on. Fried foods went off my personal menu. I also reduced my intake of saturated fat (the kind found in animal products like whole milk and bacon) and hydrogenated oils, both of which are linked to high blood cholesterol levels. With diabetes already increasing my risk of heart disease, I didn't need my diet to exacerbate the problem. I joined a gym and started exercising more. The working out part was mostly all right. I'm a former athlete, so I don't hate exercise the way some people do. But the eating was difficult; no, it was next to impossible.

When you're a food addict, it's hard to make the transition to healthy eating. Initially, I was doing okay and lost about twenty-five pounds, but I think I was still somewhat in denial. I was edging toward making healthier choices, but I was continuing to eat more than I should. After a year into it, I still had a lot of weight to lose, and I had even gained back some of the weight I had initially lost.

I wasn't the only person in my extended family battling with weight. My mother-in-law was too. When she started talking about having weight-loss surgery, I was a little surprised. It seemed kind of drastic—going under the knife is always risky. She went through with it, though, and she lost a tremendous amount of weight. It was amazing. And she's kept the weight off.

My own decision to have gastric bypass surgery wasn't an easy one. I really gave it careful consideration. Learning I had diabetes definitely threw me for a loop, and it led me to a crossroads. I wanted to get a handle on my weight once and for all and get to a place where I could really control it. And so far, let's be honest, my efforts were only mediocre. I felt I needed to do something right then and there to give me hope and make me feel as though I was capable of living a healthier life. I needed a jump start. I talked to my doctor about it, and he said, "Look, if you can't get your weight under control, having a gastric bypass is probably one of the best things you can do. It's worked for a lot of people, and you are definitely a good candidate."

By then *American Idol* had already debuted and had two hit seasons. Kelly Clarkson had been crowned the first Idol and was proving herself worthy of the mantle, with Justin Guarini nicely bringing up the rear. Then Ruben Studdard, another great artist, came along to win the second time around. Suddenly everything changed. The auditions were packed with aspiring singers. People are a little skeptical when something is brand new—we only had about 10 million viewers the first season—but *American Idol* was now a proven entity. Eventually, by Season 7's finale, we'd get 32 million people watching the show.

I'd been in the public eye before, but never with such high visibility. I'd spent most of the few years just before as a behind-the-scenes guy. Now people were coming up to me all the time. It was cool. I think what helped me take it in stride was that I already had kids. I wasn't about to go wild with newfound celebrity. And I still had my health to worry about. Season 2 was over, summer was starting, and I was on hiatus from the show, so if I wanted to do something that would require recovering at home, this was the time. I picked up the phone and called Dr. Fobi.

Mal Fobi, MD, has been performing weight-loss surgeries longer than almost anyone—since 1981. He's devoted practically his whole professional life to it, and he has developed his own specific variation on the gastric bypass called the Fobi Pouch (see "What Is a Gastric Bypass?" on page 66). That's what I had.

When you decide to have the surgery, you don't just walk into the hospital one day and say, "Okay. Let's go, dawg." They give you all kinds of tests, and you have several meetings with both a dietitian and a psychologist. It's a big step, so they want you to be well prepared—not just medically but psychologically. This is drastic; you're risking your life, and you've got to be able to be in your right mind about it. You've also got to be prepared to change your life after the surgery. That's one of the main reasons they have you talk to all these experts: not only does your head have to be in the right place so that you can cope with the changes, you need to know how to eat right and what type of exercise you should do so that you can maintain your weight loss. Once the surgery is over, the education and support continue. You're encouraged to continue counseling and to join support groups. That's helpful because nobody knows what you're going through like someone else who's had the surgery too.

One of the most important parts of my preparation for such a big undertaking was asking myself if I was going to be able to follow through on the lifestyle changes that are part of the deal. I was going to have to eat healthier foods, and far less of them. And I was going to have to commit to physical activity. That was nonnegotiable. Then, of course, as you might imagine, having a gastric bypass is not exactly a walk in the park. Any kind of surgery has the potential for tragedy, so it's not something I could undertake lightly. Some people have died while undergoing the procedure, and some of them have severe complications. Of course, most people don't. Most people come out just fine, and my decision to go through with the surgery had a lot to do with the fact that my mother-in-law had been one of them. A good friend of mine had had the procedure, too, and he was also doing well. The biggest thing for me, though, was the fact that I had type 2 diabetes, and I was desperate for any kind of help I could get to deal with the problem. I looked at surgery as a last-ditch effort.

The night before I was scheduled to go in for the procedure—it was in July 2003—Erika and I barely slept. First thing in the morning, we got in the car and drove the forty-five minutes from our home to the hospital where Dr. Fobi practices. When we got there, Erika gave me an out. She was afraid I wouldn't wake up from the surgery. "You can walk out of here right now and nobody will say anything about it." No, I was ready to go. "Bring it on," I said. "I am going to be okay."

What Is a Gastric Bypass, and Should You Have One?

Weight-loss surgery has been a great thing for me, but it's definitely not for everyone, and I don't want to make it seem like it's the only way, or even the best way, to lose weight. It's very risky: The Centers for Disease Control and Prevention reports that 10 percent of people have complications after the surgery. Other reports indicate that one in two hundred to three hundred people die. These are stats you've got to consider if you're contemplating a gastric bypass. Weight-loss surgery (or bariatric surgery, as it's often called) is the weapon of last resort.

And it's really only for some people. If you've just got

twenty or thirty pounds to lose, don't get any ideas. You've got to be at least one hundred pounds overweight to qualify for a gastric bypass. The only time a (reputable) doctor will operate on someone with less to lose is if that person has diabetes, high blood pressure, or other problems that are complicated by obesity.

It's also important to understand what it entails. A gastric bypass isn't a little nip and tuck. It's major (and it's very expensive, so keep that in mind too). There are a few different kinds of gastric bypasses, and none of them is simple.

The Roux-en-Y gastric bypass, for example, is a procedure where the stomach is stapled, creating a pouch and effectively and dramatically reducing the stomach's size. Since the pouch can only hold small amounts of food, it makes you feel full fast, so you end up consuming a lot less. The surgery also involves bypassing a part of the small intestine, which changes the way you digest everything you eat. Afterward, you won't absorb as many nutrients, including fat. To make up for lost vitamins and minerals, you need to take supplements.

Another common type of weight-loss surgery is called vertical banded gastroplasty. This is similar to the surgery I just described—a small pouch is created—but the intestines are not rerouted. This reduces the stomach's size, but it doesn't change the way you digest nutrients.

There is also a weight-loss surgery that uses no staples. It's called the LAP-BAND System. This procedure involves placing an adjustable band around the upper portion of the stomach.

Like I said, the surgery I had was a modified gastric bypass called the Fobi Pouch. This procedure doesn't use staples, either, but divides the stomach in two, reattaches it in different areas, and uses a band to keep the stomach from stretching. It makes it harder to binge, so it results in more weight loss and longer weight-loss maintenance.

As noted, this is serious business. You have to have anesthesia, and the recovery time can be weeks. It's not something to jump into. If you're thinking about a gastric bypass, get all the information you can, and give it a lot of thought.

After the surgery I spent three days in the hospital, then I went home where Taylor, Zoe, and Jordan were waiting. They were worried that the surgery would hurt. It did, but just a little bit and only for about a week. One thing I had going for me was that I had had a laparoscopic procedure, which is less invasive than the standard gastric bypass. Instead of cutting you wide open, the surgeon makes only small incisions, then does the work through a narrow, tubelike instrument. Still, it took three nail-biting hours (well, not nail-biting for me—I was totally zonked), and once it was over my stomach had only a 20 cc capacity, which is about a handful of peanuts. It also had a ring around it, and that prevents me from eating more than that handful at a time.

The results came quickly. By September I had lost 52 pounds, by October another 15. I went into a grocery store where I shop all the time, and the clerk, whom I knew well, didn't even recognize me. He asked to see my driver's license! I dropped from 329 pounds to 229 pounds, lost twelve inches off my waist, and went down five shirt sizes in a few months. Later I dropped about 25 more pounds. The greatest part about all of this, though, was that I felt so much better. I could breathe more easily, sleep well, and my energy had doubled. Just a month after the surgery, I went out with Mariah Carey on her Charmbracelet World Tour, traveling to Japan. *American Idol* auditions started up again as we embarked on Season 3, and we were about to meet one of the most gifted *Idol* winners, Fantasia Barrino. I also had a great vacation in Hawaii. Through it all, I was feeling awesome.

A gastric bypass is not like liposuction. The doctors don't remove any fat, but the reason everyone loses weight so quickly afterward is that they can't eat any solid food for about two months. You're subsisting on 500, 600, maybe 700 calories. And guess what? Anyone, no matter what size you are, is going to lose weight on so few calories. So I slimmed down fast. I was practically living on chicken broth, and I remember craving hamburgers for the first two weeks. Burgers, burgers, burgers. In-N-Out Burger burgers with mustard, mayo, ketchup, pickles—the works. It was all I could think about. Then, about three weeks into it, the craving went away. It's funny how that works. I learned a lot about myself from that little interlude. If I give something up—even if it's something I'm crazy about—then give myself some time to get used to it, I find I can live without it. That doesn't mean I never get cravings anymore. All those Southern biscuits and pies I grew up on? They're locked in my sensory memory, and I don't think I will ever entirely stop wanting them. But during those weeks when surgery limited my options, I proved to myself that cravings do diminish over time and that I could handle them.

A Conversation with Dr. Fobi

If anybody knows a thing or two about obesity and weight-loss surgery, it's my surgeon Mathias (known as Mal) Fobi, MD, medical director of the Center for Surgical Treatment of Obesity at St. Mary Medical Center in Long Beach, California. Dr. Fobi has been performing weight-loss surgery since the late seventies, though I'm sure it's something he never imagined he'd be doing as a boy growing up in Cameroon. His hometown was so small that "When we went to the city and saw streetlights," he says, "we thought they were many moons— we'd never seen electricity before." He'd never even been in a car until the drive to the airport when he left Cameroon to study in the United States.

What I like about Dr. Fobi (besides, of course, his technical skill) is that he's a realist. Despite the way he makes his livelihood, he's the first to tell you that surgery is not a panacea for obesity. I talked to him at length about the topic and here's what he had to say.

RJ: When I first talked to you about the possibility of having a gastric bypass, you were up front about what it would really mean for me.

MF: The surgery is like a car that you give somebody to transport them from one place to another. It makes the transportation easy. But, like a car, you have to maintain it. If the transmission oil is not there, the brake fluid is not there, you can't go anywhere. The car gets stuck. That's the way you have to look at the surgery. It's effective. Some people use it better than others, but some people let the car do all the work, and after a while the car runs out of oil and doesn't work.

RJ: What's one of the hardest things for people like me—people who have a pretty crazy work life—in terms of doing the maintenance?

MF: Sometimes it's hard to get people with a certain lifestyle, and people in the entertainment business fall into this category, to eat at least three times a day. You have to remember that obesity is a medical problem, so eating is like medication, and you have to take your medication regularly. The other problem is that some people eat all day long. The surgery will only work if you allow twenty minutes for lunch, dinner, and supper because in twenty minutes you can only consume so much.

RJ: Why do you think obesity is such a problem today?

MF: Most people who are obese have a genetic tendency. Let's use cars as an example again. Human beings are like cars. You have the motorcycle, a small Volkswagen, a big Mercedes-Benz, a regular truck, and a sixteen-wheeler. The sixteen-wheeler might get ten miles to the gallon, the motorcycle ninety miles per gallon, and the others in-between. You understand what I'm saying? Efficiency. Different people have different metabolic efficiency. Overweight people do not necessarily eat more than the regular-weight person. But once they are overweight, they cannot do many things and therefore tend to eat more and put on more weight.

RJ: It's hard to exercise when you're carrying a lot of weight.

MF: Yes. And as society becomes more sedentary, more and more people are being recruited to obesity. The incidence of obesity is growing all over the world because more and more people are now using automobiles. And right now robotics and computers are doing everything. Another reason is the easy availability of food—and oversizing. Portions are double and triple sized. Also, eating is a pleasure response. In America we entertain with the mouth. You walk into someone's office or home, and he or she offers you a cup of coffee. You get some cookies, peanuts. So you're going to eat, and when you eat and you have this genetic predisposition you're going to put on weight.

RJ: What about emotional problems. Do you think people eat too much because of emotional problems?

MF: If you're depressed and you sit around and eat a lot, you're going to gain more weight. But that part has been overplayed. Fat *causes* emotional problems. When you see people who are overweight, they often do not think of themselves first. They always come second. They're the ones that arrange the party in the office, and they're the ones who do the care giving. They put themselves second because of lack of self-esteem.

When you are overweight and you walk into a room, people are looking at you. You go to a brunch buffet and you get a plate, and people are looking at what you have on it. The person next to you might have double what you have on your plate, but no one is going to be paying attention if that person is thin. That has to affect the overweight person psychologically. If you are overweight, people think you should not eat. If you're five foot eight and 140 pounds, you can go fill your plate. You get praised for eating. The patients who come for surgery aren't looking to be handsome. They're not trying to be beautiful. They just want to walk into a room and not be noticed, like everyone else. They just want to live a normal life.

RJ: When I had the surgery, I had to really think about it and ask myself if I was committed to doing the work to keep the weight off. How do you tell if someone is ready?

MF: It is the responsibility of the individual to follow the therapy after surgery. But it also demonstrates some of the prejudice in society when those individuals are asked about their commitment to staying with it. If someone walks in with a lump in her breast, then has surgery, am I going to ask her if she will be committed to coming for chemotherapy afterward? No. Obesity is also a medical problem.

RJ: Well, the thing about commitment is that it's just so much easier to do the things you need to do to stay healthy when you feel better.

MF: It's like being born again. It's like seeing a young lady who comes from a poor family and she's helping her mom in the restaurant, cooking in the back. Suddenly Randy Jackson and his crew find this girl, and she can sing. Now they put a little bit of makeup on her, give her a microphone, and she becomes a big star. We all have the natural potential, and we need the right exposure to make us bloom. The surgery is a tool to help someone bloom.

———

The weight I lost right after the surgery was what you might call the first phase of change. It's funny that Dr. Fobi used the metaphor of a flower blooming when talking about how contestants on *American Idol* and people who are trying to win the weight-loss battle have something in common: it's a metaphor I often use too. What really impresses me more than anything about some of these kids is how they grow. To some extent they do it while they're on the show, but some of them—Kelly Clarkson, Carrie Underwood, Clay Aiken, Jordin Sparks, to name a few—continue to blossom once they've moved on. Some of this can be attributed to their success, but to me it's also based on their growth as people. They're the ones who seem to stay grounded and grow spiritually, to gain confidence and be true to themselves. One thing *American Idol* does is give these artists a shot, a chance to jump into the ring. How well they ultimately do depends on how good they are at seizing the opportunity.

When you have a gastric bypass, you're also given a shot, but it's up to you to make the most of it. So in the first phase after the surgery, I lost a lot of weight. Now, how was I going to capitalize on it? First, I had to move into the next postsurgical phase: learning to live with a stomach so drastically reduced in size that you simply cannot eat too much without suffering some nasty consequences. I now have to chew every bite really, really well or the food gets stuck and makes me throw up or feel like I have heartburn. It seems like I can't breathe and I start to gag. When it happens, I just decide, "This eating thing is closed for now." I don't even want to think about eating because it's such a terrible feeling.

Because I can't handle as much food at one time, I now eat lots of small meals instead of three big ones. The particular procedure I had also changed the way I process food so that I absorb less protein and fat. And I can't eat anything too sweet or rich, or I experience something known as dumping. Dumping is this weird phenomenon that affects people who've had a gastric bypass. On occasion, if you eat the wrong thing (it can be different for different people), food "dumps" into your intestine without being digested, and your body, in essence, throws water at it to try to dilute the food. The result is that you feel awful—all dizzy, nauseous, sweaty, and weak. Sometimes your heart may even race. Dumping is like nothing I've ever known before, and I try to avoid it all costs. That means that some of the foods I always loved, like peanut butter and a few different kinds of chocolate, are off my regular menu.

What I haven't mentioned yet, but which is really the heart and soul of the whole gastric bypass matter, is that after the surgery my diabetes went into remission. My blood sugar returned to a normal level. Losing weight was great, but going off diabetes medication was like hitting it out of the park, baby! Recently, I heard that in three-quarters of the people who have the surgery, diabetes completely disappears. Gone. It can even happen in a matter of days, before much weight is gone. This is probably because the surgery changes the way food moves through your system, lowering blood glucose levels. Then, as you begin to lose weight, it helps further because excess body fat can create insulin resistance; once the fat comes off, the insulin resistance resolves. This is one of those cases where you say to yourself, "You know what? Those darned doctors may know something!" Lost the weight, off the oral medication, blood sugar back to a normal level.

Okay, but this wasn't the end of it. I still had phase three to contend with: maintenance. This is what everyone thinks is the easy part because, after all, you've got physical limitations now. Your stomach is smaller so you feel fuller faster, you're not absorbing all your calories, and the hormones that send hunger messages to the brain may even be diminished because of the way your digestive system has been reworked. But while that's all true, it doesn't mean that you can't screw up. Plenty of people do.

Here's the thing. While my body was giving me different signals than it ever had before, I still had to do the work not to override those signals. How many times have you said, "I'm so full, I couldn't eat another thing," then the dessert cart rolls around and you're like, "I'll have the crème brûlée"? Physiological signals can be ignored *even when you've had a gastric bypass.*

By changing your physiology, a gastric bypass sets up new rules for you, but you can break those rules. It doesn't feel good, and I know because I've done it on occasion. But it can be done. Eventually, you can just kind of "eat through" your reconfigured anatomy and end up back where you started: fat all over again. Maybe you've heard about people who have had a gastric bypass but gained back all the weight. It's not because the surgery didn't work; it's because they chose, for whatever reason, not to do the work needed to maintain the results.

So surgery was not going to be a guarantee for me. It put me way down the field; it was a great jump start and I'm glad I did it. But in some ways it's like going on a diet and losing a lot of weight. It's a Band-Aid. I couldn't go back to my old ways of eating instantly, like I did when I went off diets in the past, but I could have eventually worked my way back to those bad habits. Plus, while a gastric bypass may help you with your eating, it doesn't *make* you move your body, and movement is a really important piece of the puzzle—for keeping off weight *and* for lowering blood sugar. Now, that said, when you lose a lot of weight, moving is a whole lot easier. A thousand million percent easier. So some people who were very sedentary before a gastric bypass will automatically start to move more. But that's incidental. Ultimately, after the anesthesia wore off, I still awoke from my surgery to the problem of how to keep the weight off. (We'll talk more about exercise in chapter 7.)

One thing I had in my favor was that I was highly motivated. In the span of about a year and a half I had discovered that I had a deadly disease, and I had undergone major surgery. These are the kinds of things that shake you up and make you truly want to change. My mission after the gastric bypass was to find ways to keep eating well and to increase the amount of exercise I was doing. In that way I was (and am) like anyone else who struggles with his or her weight. Again, shrinking your body size isn't really the battle; it's keeping the weight off. Eventually, I did come up with a plan that would keep me from backsliding. I changed my life. That's what I want to talk about next.

Real-Life Alert
How to Be a Good Dinner Guest
(Without Overeating)

Have you ever gone to dinner at someone's home, only to be slightly horrified when they bring out the double-cheese lasagna followed by the chocolate mousse for dessert? Delicious as it may be, you can feel your arteries clogging and your butt expanding as you politely swallow forkful after forkful, trying not to offend your host.

I've been at dinner parties where people on diets have brought their own food. My feeling is, you gotta do what you gotta do, but I have a different approach. Instead, I try to sample everything in small portions, and if there is one dish that seems healthier than the rest, I'll focus on that. I've trained my eyes, mind, and soul to look for the healthy option. *I'll have a bowl of salad, a small square of lasagna, and a few bites of dessert—thank you very much.* How can any host be offended by that? Besides, I've got more than someone's feelings to worry about; I've got my health to think of. This is my guiding principle.

And I will admit that it's sometimes easier to abide by that principle in theory than in reality. It can be hard to have just a smidgen of lasagna and bite of dessert when everyone else at the table is tossing back wine and indulging freely. I'm not immune to the temptation, and I'm sure neither are you. But here are two other things to bear in mind. First, if you do decide to throw caution to the wind, don't abandon all mindfulness. Listen to your body and see if you really do need to eat all that's on your plate (see page 101 for more about monitoring your satiety). You don't have to finish all your food just because it's there or you think it would be rude not to.

Second, enjoy yourself. Relish the meal and the time with friends, then *immediately* return to your regular healthy habits. Don't pig out over the rest of the weekend because you feel as though you've already blown it. What would have happened if David Cook sang a hip-hop song, got bad commentary (because he is so obviously *not* a hip-hop dude), then came back week after week singing hip-hop songs? Disaster. One hip-hop song wouldn't have done much damage to his chances, but a string of them would have. Likewise, one big meal isn't going to do much damage to your body, but a string of them will.

Spaghetti Squash with Spicy Meatballs in Tomato Sauce

I made a dish similar to this with Martha Stewart on her show, and I've been digging it ever since. Eating spaghetti squash rather than regular pasta is a good way to lower your carb intake, and this version tastes a lot like old-fashioned spaghetti and meatballs.

Serves 6

Have on hand:
9 × 13 inch baking dish
aluminum foil
medium and large mixing bowls
10-inch skillet with lid

1 spaghetti squash, about 2½ pounds
1 cup fresh bread crumbs
⅓ cup evaporated skim milk
2½ cups marinara sauce, good quality
⅓ cup red wine
2 teaspoons ground cumin, divided
1¼ teaspoons ground cinnamon
¼ teaspoon cayenne, divided
⅛ teaspoon ground cloves
1 pound ground turkey breast
½ cup finely chopped fresh parsley, divided

freshly ground black pepper, to taste
½ teaspoon salt (optional)

Preheat oven to 375°F.

Slice squash in half vertically, scoop out seeds, and place cut side down in a 9 × 13 inch baking dish. Add enough water to create a depth of ¼ inch. Cover with foil and bake 45 minutes. Remove from oven and keep covered.

Combine bread crumbs and evaporated milk in a medium mixing bowl; set aside.

Put marinara sauce in a 10-inch skillet over medium-high heat. Stir in wine, 1 teaspoon cumin, cinnamon, ⅛ teaspoon cayenne, and cloves. Bring to a boil. Reduce heat, cover, and simmer.

In a large bowl, mash bread crumbs into a smooth paste. Add turkey, remaining cumin and cayenne, ¼ cup parsley, and black pepper to taste (if sodium is not an issue, add the salt). Mix with your hands until well combined. Wetting hands to keep from sticking, roll mixture into about thirty 1½-inch meatballs. Carefully lower meatballs into simmering sauce. Cover and cook 15 minutes. Uncover and stir in remaining parsley.

Using a fork, scrape the strands of squash from the shell and onto a platter or into a bowl. Serve squash hot with meatballs and sauce spooned on top.

Per serving: *187 calories, 4 g fat (18.8% calories from fat), 20 g protein, 16 g carbohydrate, 2 g dietary fiber, 43 mg cholesterol, 653 mg sodium.*

NOLA Red Beans and Rice

New Orleans is famous for its fattier fare, but once in a while we Louisianans eat something simple like this beans and rice dish. Of course back home it's often made with some kind of pork fat, but believe me it tastes just as terrific with the unhealthy fat left out.

Serves 6

Have on hand:
large skillet with lid

1 tablespoon canola oil
1 cup finely chopped onion
¾ cup finely chopped green bell pepper
½ cup finely chopped celery
3 cloves garlic, minced
1 cup converted rice
2½ cups fat-free chicken broth
2 teaspoons salt-free Cajun spice blend (see recipe on page 16)
2 cans (15 oz) low-sodium kidney beans, drained and rinsed

Heat oil in a large skillet over medium-high heat. Add onion, green pepper, celery, and garlic and sauté until vegetables are soft. Add rice and continue to sauté until rice becomes opaque, about 5 minutes. Stir in broth and seasoning and bring to a boil. Reduce heat to simmer, cover, and cook 15 minutes. Stir in beans, cover, and cook 5 minutes, or until liquid is absorbed.

Per serving: *235 calories, 3 g fat (9.7% calories from fat), 12 g protein, 44 g carbohydrate, 7 g dietary fiber, 0 mg cholesterol, 293 mg sodium.*

CHAPTER FIVE

Eating with a New Attitude

A fter a lifetime of struggling continually with weight and food, I can't tell you how good it feels to sit down at a table, select what I'm going to eat, and know that I made the right choice. It's effortless. Easy. I don't fight with myself anymore. In the old days, it was like I had a devil on one shoulder and an angel on the other, and they were constantly bickering.

Have the fried chicken.
If you do, you're going to hate yourself in the morning.
Order the spinach salad with low-calorie dressing instead.
How boring!

I felt like I could never win. Either I was going to eat something completely sinful and feel guilty about it, or I was going to eat something totally unsatisfying and be disappointed. There was no middle ground, and most of the time whichever choice I made would lead me to take in too many calories, if not at first, then later on. If I had the fried chicken, well, that speaks for itself. That's just fattening. If I had the spinach salad with low-calorie dressing, I might feel virtuous for a while, but I would end up raiding the refrigerator later that night because I felt so cheated. Or because I thought I "earned" it.

Things aren't like that for me anymore. Most of the time—because that's what I'm going for, a good, not a perfect, record—I can look at a menu or open up my cupboards at home and make a choice that will both satisfy me and keep me healthy. It's not a big deal anymore. Eating wisely comes naturally now. If you told me this five years ago, I wouldn't have believed you. Not a guy who lived for a mess of ribs smothered in barbecue sauce with a colossal-sized piece of red velvet cake for dessert. Yet here I am, eating healthfully and, most surprisingly, happily, just about every day.

While it's pretty easy for me now, I don't want to give you the impression that it didn't take a lot of work to get to this point or that I never have a day when I don't want to throw out the rules, toss back a peach Nehi, and sink my teeth into a MoonPie. Sometimes I really, really want to—but I don't. As I have said, I grew up on sweets with a master baker (my mom) in the house. So as you might imagine, finding out that I had diabetes and that I had to cut way back on sugar was like, whoa, hit me where it hurts. And that was just one of the changes I had to make. It took time, energy, and a lot of effort to relearn how to eat.

I'm sure I don't have to tell you that to lose weight and keep it off you have to eat fewer calories and exercise (more on exercise coming up, by the way). The two go hand in hand. However, I'd like to add another component to the formula: exercise, eat fewer calories, *and* eat more healthfully. Because this isn't just about weight; it's about health too. You don't hear much about people overeating carrots and broccoli. If you're overeating, usually that heap of foods includes ones that either clog your arteries or have no redeeming nutritional value. You know what I'm talking about. All the cinnamon rolls and cupcakes. Sodas, bagels slathered with cream cheese, potato chips, and onion rings. They've got calories galore (and probably lots of saturated and trans fats too) but not many vitamins, minerals, phytochemicals, or fiber—all the things that science now tells us help prevent disease. Your goal should be, not only to eat less, but to eat *better*. That combination of fewer calories and more-nutritious foods is going to help ensure your well-being and make you feel good too.

It's funny. I went for years eating nothing but junk without even realizing that it was making me feel lethargic and depleted. Once you change your diet and start eating more fruits and vegetables, whole grains, and lean proteins, it's amazing how much more energetic you feel. But it's not all that surprising. You're finally giving your body the food it needs—it's got to have some impact on how you feel. And I tell you what, it's also going to have an impact on your numbers: blood sugar, cholesterol, triglycerides. So don't just think about reducing the quantity of food, think about a higher quality of food.

I'm sure you know which foods are healthy and which ones are not, and if you don't, get yourself a nutrition book and find out. This chapter isn't about that. Erin Naimi, a registered dietitian with a lot of experience counseling people who struggle with their weight, is going to comment on some particular foods and food myths, but the bulk of this chapter is devoted to strategies that will help you make good choices, eat fewer calories, and, as a result, lose the weight that may be endangering your health.

The important thing to note about these strategies is that you can't just use them for a couple of weeks. Diets have a beginning and an end, but the way of eating I'm talking about—healthfully and moderately, but without denying yourself all of life's gastronomic pleasures—is something you do for life. It requires commitment, but I know you can do it, dawg. Commitment is hot! Eating wisely is hot! Good health is hot!

What Is the Reality of You?

Typically, when you go on a diet you begin by following a prescribed regimen. This time you're not going on a diet and there's no prescription for you to follow, so don't start worrying about what you're going to eat (or not going to eat) just yet. Instead, start by thinking about your life. How do you go about your day? What are the demands of your schedule? What are your social, professional, and family lives like? In other words, what is the reality of you? These questions are going to let you see your patterns, and that will help you make adaptations that you'll be able to live with. On page 121, I talk about keeping a food journal, something that really helped me see the mistakes I was making. Before you try writing down everything you're eating, you might try writing down your complete schedule for two weeks to see what your regular patterns are. Here's a typical day in my life late in the *Idol* season.

8:00 a.m. Wake up. Hit the treadmill for thirty minutes.

9:00 a.m. Bowl of oatmeal with some berries and a cup of coffee for breakfast.

9:30 a.m. In the car and on my way to the office.

10:00 a.m. Check in with my assistant to see what's up for the day, make and take about fifty phone calls.

11:00 a.m. Meeting with singer I might produce. Just enough time to nibble on an energy bar.

12:00 p.m. Order in for lunch: chicken sandwich and bowl of asparagus soup. More phone calls.

1:00 p.m. Back in the car and on my way to the *Idol* set.

1:30 p.m. Greet everyone. It's a very cordial environment. Maybe check out the dress rehearsal, maybe not. I really prefer to judge the performances in the moment. I usually don't take a second look at the singers on tape at home either.

2:30 p.m. Time for a briefing on what's going to be happening on the show that day—any changes in timing or schedule, special guests, and so on. There's really not very much prep for the show. It's one of the few *real* reality shows on the air. There is no script. We just go and do it.

3:00 p.m. Get a little love from the hair, makeup, and wardrobe people.

4:00 p.m. Have a snack of vegetables and dip and a little turkey from the backstage buffet. Try to avoid the cookie platter.

5:00 p.m. We're live! (As you might know, the show is live, East Coast time, during the later part of the season and prerecorded in the earlier portion. Early in the season, my schedule is also more demanding since we've got more performances to watch and more shows to do.)

6:00 p.m. That's a wrap, and I'm out of there. What I do next is variable. Ryan, Simon, and I have a "boys club"; we like to hang out, so sometimes we'll go to dinner after the show, occasionally inviting some of the Fox or Fremantle executives along. Paula is always welcome too. She's a real girl, but we love her, so we let her crash the boys club when she's in the mood. If I'm not hanging with my colleagues, and don't have a dinner meeting, then as soon as the show's over I'll split and go home to eat with my family. It's not quite Ozzie and Harriet, but it's a far cry from the days when quitting time was 3:00 a.m. and I'd be heading for the closest chicken-and-waffle joint.

I'm not a big believer in making over your life to suit your dietary needs. That's because it almost never works. It's easy to con yourself into thinking that you're never going to find yourself in a fast-food restaurant, or that you aren't going to hang out with your friends on the weekends because they like to break out the chips and dip, or that you're not going to get home late from work and want to eat something. Whatever your life is like, you've got to be honest with yourself. If these situations are your reality, you probably aren't going to change them much—but you *can* change how you handle them.

I spend a lot of time in recording studios and on the sets of TV shows, and there are always all kinds of junk food around. The other day I was on the set of my other show, *Randy Jackson Presents America's Best Dance Crew,* and there must have been nine thousand cupcakes backstage (and I mean, man, they had every kind imaginable, all from the trendiest, übercupcake place in LA). What am I going to do? Not go onto the set of a show I produce or give up working in recording studios? Of course not. What I had to do was figure out a way to cope with having all that enticing food around me. Most of the time what I do now is make sure there's something there that I *can* eat. I'm going to be a lot less tempted by nine thousand cupcakes if I can call up the deli around the corner and order a turkey sandwich (and that's what I did). If I just tried to tough it out without eating anything, I probably would have failed to keep my hands off a cupcake. Just like you might have trouble passing up the doughnuts and coffee at a workplace meeting if you didn't have something else to turn to. (And if you don't have a deli around the corner, that's when you pull one of the snacks on page 142 out of your desk drawer.)

Even though I was motivated to get healthy after finding out that I had diabetes, I wasn't motivated to change what you might call the foundation of my life: my work, my family life, my social life. I couldn't live in a convent where there would never be doughnuts or desserts or macaroni with eighteen cheeses (I exaggerate, but you know some of those mac 'n' cheese dishes are deadly). So I said to myself, "Okay, I've got to meet this head on and make smarter, better choices." Because what's the point of being healthy if you're not happy? That's just not me. I am all about living a big, full life. My schedule is crazy; I'm working all the time.

Maybe that's why I failed at dieting so many times. Most diets don't take into account that you live in the real world. They're not created with the idea that you're going to go out for dinner a lot. They don't accommodate the fact that you're going to have to eat on the run while you're driving your kids from activity to activity, or that you're going to want something to eat when you're at a basketball game. They may not offer ways to help you on those many nights when you don't have the time (or inclination) to cook dinner.

I also found that some diets are so rigid that they leave you hanging during those times when your energy starts to flag. Everyone seems to crash at some point during the day. One talent agency I've visited even has someone come around with an ice cream sundae cart in the afternoons to make sure its personnel aren't sleeping on the job. I'm not saying that having an ice cream cart in your office is the real world—this is Hollywood—but you know what I'm talking about. How many times have you run out for a megacalorie latte or candy bar when that afternoon slump hits?

If you're going to change how you eat for good—not just for a few weeks but forever—then you have to find a way to work healthy eating into the life you lead. Here's an example. Most people in the music business have partying in their blood, and I'm no exception. There's always a bunch of parties after the Grammy Awards (I don't even go to the show now; I just hit the parties). Some are in ballrooms at hotels like the Mondrian in Hollywood; some are at hot restaurants of the moment. Some, like one hosted by *Details* magazine, are at private estates. Now that I'm on *Idol*, I get invited to all these TV, movie, and fund-raising parties too. Things like Ellen DeGeneres's fiftieth birthday party (fun—and funny) and post-Emmy soirees.

I can still party with the best of them, but by that I mean I have a good time. I'm not drinking anymore, and I'm not pigging out. What I do instead is concentrate on the best part of a party: the people. What I used to do was just eat mindlessly while talking. A guy would come around with a plate of fritters, and I'd grab one just because they were there. Or I'd stand next to the table with the cheese and crackers and go for it, never thinking about what I was doing. Again, the food was there.

But once I began to get serious about regaining my health, I tried a different tack. I paid attention to the fact that I often really wasn't that hungry, so I didn't just pick up food and drink automatically. If I'm really hungry, then, yeah, I'll allow myself an hors d'oeuvre or two, but mostly I get something like a sparkling water to keep my hands and mouth occupied. Then I focus on catching up with old friends or chatting with new people. After all, aren't conversation and all the off-the-wall things that people say (and sometimes do) what partying is really about?

Another tactic I try these days is to eat before I go. That way I know I'm going to be a lot less tempted to follow the hors d'oeuvre server around the room. I'd rather sit there and have a meal in a controlled eating environment (like my home or office) than stand around snatching finger foods off a tray. The latter could spell disaster. And that's not what I'm into anymore. I strive to be a conscious eater.

What I'm urging you to do is to turn the traditional idea of a diet on its head. Don't start out by saying, "Okay, I have to eat these particular foods at this particular time of day so my life will have to change to accommodate them." Start out by saying, "Okay, this is my life, now how can I make better choices and when I do eat some of my favorite foods, eat less of them?" I'm not asking you to change where you go, who you hang out with, or how you spend your time. I'm just asking you to change some of what you typically eat and how much of it you consume. Believe me, this is an easier way to lose weight than rewriting your whole life.

For me it works something like this. I'm home for breakfast, so that's easy. I just keep the right stuff in my house. I might have oatmeal with chopped Asian pear stirred in, or an egg white omelet. I change it around so I don't get bored. If I'm having lunch with someone whose record I might produce? That's cool. I have scoped out the restaurants near my office, and I know which ones will have something healthy I can eat, or if their food is a little higher in calories than I'd like, at least it can be ordered in small portions (this is where I might choose an appetizer instead of an entrée). I'm big on small portions—we all desperately need portion control.

Sometimes I'll be working through the dinner hour, but it's not a problem. I make sure I have a protein bar or shake to tide me over so I'm not tempted to pull over to the 7-Eleven for a bag of chips on my way home. Sometimes you just have to put some gas in the tank, of course, but if you ate an energy bar or other healthy snack an hour or so earlier—even if it's not the perfect meal—it will be much easier to avoid heading inside for that bag of chips.

There are a billion solutions out there. You've just got to plan for the situations you know you're going to find yourself in.

Learn What It Feels Like to Be Truly Hungry—and Comfortably Full

When my kids were very young, they would ask for food when they were hungry and just naturally stop eating when they were full. They didn't seem to need to finish all the food on their plates or in their little snack cups just because it was there. I probably was the same way when I was a kid, but after years of eating beyond the point of fullness, that natural pattern was lost to me. Of course, it didn't help that in my household not finishing your food was an insult to the cook. Plus the general vibe was that if food is available, you'd be crazy not to eat it—and eat all of it. Every culture has its own way of guilt-tripping kids into finishing what's on their plates, training them to eat beyond the point of natural satisfaction. If it isn't "don't insult the cook," it's "don't you know there are children starving in Africa?"

What I've discovered during my journey to good health is that learning to listen to your body is *the* most important step along the way. You don't have to count calories or weigh and measure your food if you pay attention to your internal barometer. If you eat when you're hungry (and by that I mean physically hungry, not craving food because you're bored or depressed) and stop when you're full (not stuffed to the gills), then you're going to eat less and lose weight.

Getting to this point was a real process for me. I had been ignoring the signals my body was sending for so long that I didn't really even know what it meant to be full. Stuffed, yes, because I would often eat past the stage of being pleasantly full to the stage of feeling like a balloon about to burst. But as I've said, where I come from that was considered a good way to feel.

On the flip side of that, I didn't really know what it felt like to have a normal level of hunger either. Oh, I knew what it felt like to be famished, because I'd often let myself get to that point of no return. Since I'm a mad, crazy, busy person and have been since I was fourteen years old, I would often forget about eating for hours on end. No breakfast, no lunch. Then, of course, I'd be so hungry I'd eat like a racehorse. I asked Erin about it.

"When you go throughout your day ignoring your hunger signals, your body can't trust that it's going to be fed at regular intervals, so of course when food becomes available you end up overeating and ignoring signs of fullness," she says. And it's not just that I would eat too much; I would also make awful choices. When you're famished, all good judgment goes out the window and it becomes a lot easier to justify sitting down to a plate of macaroni and cheese at midnight.

The other thing I used to do all the time was eat more out of habit than out of true hunger. I'm sure there were many times I devoured a whole meal when my stomach was already full. I'd go out for dinner, and because it was expected, I'd order an appetizer, entrée, and dessert—even though I might have eaten something like a big bowl of frozen yogurt just an hour before. (And why did I eat the frozen yogurt an hour before dinner? In an emergency effort to keep myself from crashing because—you guessed it—I hadn't bothered to eat breakfast or lunch during the day.) So that is how it would go. I'd keep ping-ponging back and forth between eating because I was ravenous and eating because it was an automatic, mindless reflex. Oh, how things have changed!

I had to change. The first reason was because I came to understand that as a diabetic it was imperative that I keep my blood sugar level on an even keel. (Normal blood sugar before eating is 90 to 130 mg/dl; normal after eating is below 180 mg/dl.) You just can't stay balanced when you go for hours and hours without eating or when you stuff yourself at one sitting. The second reason was that after my gastric bypass surgery I could no longer eat large amounts of food in one sitting, so skipping meals and then trying to make up for them with one big binge wasn't going to cut it anymore.

At first listening to, then obeying, my body's hunger and satiety signals was not easy. I wasn't used to it, and I ended up sick more than a few times. But eventually I got used to taking a moment to get a read on how I was feeling. I know I'm genuinely hungry when my energy level starts to drop. It might be different for you. Some people feel it when their stomach starts to growl or they get a little light-headed. I also no longer use an empty plate to tell me when I'm done with a meal. I eat slowly and stop along the way to get a register on whether my stomach feels full and if my energy level has returned. If it has, that's when I stop eating.

Ultimately, that means I eat less food. Yesterday, for instance, I was in the studio, and I ordered a turkey melt sandwich with a little side salad. I ate half the sandwich and felt perfectly satisfied. Before, I wouldn't have been happy unless I had the whole sandwich, the salad, and two or three other things besides. I wouldn't have stopped at half a sandwich. But now, because I listen to what's going on with my body, a half sandwich is enough. I've retrained myself.

These days, in fact, I'm so in tune with my body that I can feel whether my blood sugar is too high or too low, without even having to check it; it's like an alarm going off. I do, however, still use my blood sugar monitor once or sometimes twice a day, just out of habit. Diabetics monitor their blood sugar to figure out whether they can afford to eat something— usually a food rich in carbohydrates—or whether their blood sugar level is already too high. (It's also a way to find out how your body reacts to different types of foods. If, for instance, you want to know if a low-sugar muffin is really as good a choice as it seems, you check your blood sugar after eating it.)

The cool thing is that you don't need a medical issue like diabetes or a band around your stomach to get in touch with your body's hunger and satiety signals. Your body is trying to tell you when it's had enough, so listen up!

The first thing you need to be is mindful. As I mentioned above, the signal to stop eating is going to come from your body, not an empty plate. Sometimes you might clean your plate, but that needs to be because you are still genuinely hungry, not because you have the voice of your mother or anyone else running through your head reminding you of less-fortunate people.

Learning to recognize when your body is telling you it's had enough does take some practice. Erin advises beginning this way: Put your fork down between bites and check in with yourself. Ask yourself, "How do I feel? Do I need that second scoop of ice cream?" Well, sure, you could eat that second scoop, and probably even a third and fourth, but is your body—your *body*, not your mind—really asking for it?

The only way you're going to be able to hear what your body is saying is to slow way down and be mindful of what's going on. If you're just shoveling food into your mouth as quickly as you can, it's like being tone deaf. You're not going to get it. And it's hard to be mindful if you're eating while you're driving or carrying on a phone conversation or distracted by the TV. That's why it's so much better if you can eat without doing ten other things at the same time. Sometimes I might find myself talking to someone during a meal, and because I'm concentrating on the conversation, it's hard to listen to my body. But even if you're in a situation where you're, say, at a dinner party and involved in three conversations at once, you need to have the wherewithal to periodically turn your attention inward and savor your food so that it registers. You're not going to need double portions if the portion you just ate rang your bell. And once it has, ask yourself, "Do I feel full?" Get your answer, then obey it. Don't go trying to override the message: "Oh, but this is my favorite pasta. Who knows when I'll have it again." Of course you'll have it again. If you really want it, you can have it next week. Honor what your body is telling you.

It can help, says Erin, if you have a specific idea of what it means to be appropriately hungry and full, which is why she gives all her clients a copy of the Hunger and Satiety Evaluation Scale (see box on page 101). The scale begins at 1: starving, dizzy, insatiable and ends at 10: stuffed to the point of feeling sick. "You never want to be at a 10 or a 1," says Erin. "I encourage people to stop at 6 or 7, when they're comfortably full, and to eat when they hit a 4 or 3, just beginning to feel hungry or when the physical signs of hunger are present."

It's important to respect both sides of the coin by not only stopping when you're full but eating when you're hungry. If you've been on a hundred diets, like me, you get used to the idea that anytime you can resist the urge to eat, you're doing well. But that's not really true, because ignoring your hunger just sets you off on a roller-coaster ride, ending with you tunneling through a bag of chips while you wait for your (large) frozen pizza to come out of the oven. Satisfy your hunger when it's calling out to you, listen to your stomach when it says "That's it!" and you'll make great strides toward losing weight and improving your health.

The Hunger and Satiety Evaluation Scale

10: Stuffed to the point of feeling sick
9: Uncomfortably full; you feel stuffed
8: Very full; you've overeaten
7: Comfortably full and satisfied
6: Comfortably full, though not quite satisfied
5: Neutral, neither hungry nor full
4: Beginning signs of hunger
3: Hungry; physical signs are present and you're ready to eat
2: Very hungry; irritable and unable to concentrate
1: Starving, dizzy, insatiable

There's one caveat I'll add here. I'm really sensitive to my hunger and fullness signals now—though it took me a long time to get here—but there are people who hardly ever feel full or whose signals are really delayed. If your hunger signals don't come in loud and clear until it's too late, then I'll tell you what I tell musicians (and often *Idol* contestants) who are missing the mark: practice, practice, practice. Keep eating slowly, and always stop and wait awhile before putting seconds on your plate. If you need to, eat in a place where there is less commotion and you can listen to your body. Think, too, about what fullness really means. You may not feel the sense of satisfaction you get when you're stuffed, but you may find that once the edge is off your hunger and you feel comfortable, you can live with it. Be patient too. Just as you used to be in the habit of eating until you were overly full, you'll develop a new habit of eating until you feel contentedly full. It will come naturally to you.

Food Myths: Let's Set the Record Straight

Living in Los Angeles, a town where people like to talk about food, weight loss, and nutrition, I hear so many different things about what to eat and what not to eat that it sometimes makes my head spin. What's myth, I always wonder, and what's truth? As a registered dietitian, Erin Naimi has heard just about everything (to learn more about her experience, see page xxx). Erin and I sat down to talk about what's fact and what's fiction.

RJ: Okay, coffee. Thumbs up or thumbs down?

EN: Coffee is fine, but you have to consider a few things about caffeine. Caffeine is an appetite suppressant, so initially it may inhibit your hunger. But caffeine also causes blood sugar levels to plummet. A lot of people use coffee as their only breakfast, so the fact that they're already on empty means that they may experience a pretty steep drop in blood sugar. That can make you very shaky and panicky. It can also make you want to eat to get rid of the feeling.

RJ: After the gastric bypass I found out that coffee, because it's a diuretic, was depleting my potassium level, so I stopped drinking so much and now I only have one cup a day. And it's fine.

EN: One to two cups a day isn't a problem for most people.

RJ: One thing I've always wondered is if I don't eat as much, will my stomach shrink? Well, maybe not mine, because I've already had a gastric bypass, but will the average person's stomach shrink when given less food?

EN: If you're constantly putting excessive amounts of food into your stomach, it will stretch. It's a muscle. If you start to back off, sure, your stomach will shrink back to a certain degree. The smaller your stomach is, the faster you will get full, but having your stomach shrink back to normal size is only going to be helpful if you're listening to your body's hunger signals.

RJ: What's one of the most common misconceptions you hear from people?

EN: That there are good and bad foods, and that sugar, being a bad food, automatically turns into fat.

RJ: Does it?

EN: Food, any kind of food, whether it's a carbohydrate—and sugar is a simple form of carbohydrate—protein, or fat, is only stored as body fat when you eat more calories than your body needs to operate. When you have a piece of chocolate or a doughnut, alarms don't sound and say, "Send to butt" or "Send to hips." You have a brain to feed, muscles to fuel, as well as many other processes that require energy. All these things must be taken care of before your body stores sugar or any other types of calories as fat.

RJ: Okay, here's another one for you. Patient goes into a nutritionist's office and says, "I know I'm hot, and I want to be even hotter; that is, I want to be a smaller size. So I'm going to start with a two-week fast. I'm going to carry around this concoction made of lemon juice, cayenne pepper, and honey and drink it at my desk at work, at friends' homes, everywhere." Is that okay?

EN: I don't think it's the end of the world when somebody fasts, but I don't recommend it for several reasons. During the two weeks that you are on that diet, your body is going to be completely deprived of vital macronutrients such as protein and fat, as well as vitamins and minerals. You're not going to be getting much carbohydrate from the small amount of lemon juice and honey you're taking in either. In other words, you're not going to be getting many nutrients at all.

Being able to fast for two weeks can give you a sense of strength and willpower. "I've been able to do this," you say to yourself. But that adrenaline high is going to wear off and your body's self-protective survival mechanism will kick in. At some point, you're going to see something that you're not supposed to be eating, like a piece of bread, and give in to it. Now you're going to feel like a failure, and it all falls apart. So not only are you now in a malnourished state, you're at risk for bingeing and overeating because you're starved.

RJ: Right. Even if you lost ten or twelve pounds, you still have to come back to some sort of normalcy, right? And that's where the problems begin.

EN: You're in no better place to navigate your way through the world of food around you. You may even be more confused.

RJ: Vegetarian? Vegan? I was a vegetarian for ten years when I was involved in an Eastern science-of-the-mind religion. Break it down for us. What's the best way to go?

EN: It depends on your body, and I don't mean your blood type or anything like that. Listen to your body. If you're having dreams about a steak, then go have a piece of meat. In terms of good health, you can eat healthfully on both a vegetarian and a vegan diet, but it's a myth to think that those diets are more healthful than other types of diets. You can be a vegetarian and develop anemia and/or osteoporosis. It's not that common, but it's possible if you're not getting enough iron or calcium. And it's a little more challenging to get protein as a vegetarian or vegan, but it certainly can be done. Soy, dairy products, nuts, beans, and legumes are all excellent sources of vegetarian protein.

RJ: Will you be thinner on a vegetarian or vegan diet?
EN: Not necessarily. That's a myth too. No matter what type

of diet you follow, what matters is your ability to feed your body appropriately for its unique needs. If lacto-ovo vegetarians (who eat dairy products and eggs) and vegans (who consume no animal by-products) are mindful of their nutritional needs, they may be at a nutritional advantage compared to their omnivorous counterparts because they tend to eat more vegetables and less saturated fat. However, some vegetarians replace meat with too many carbohydrates or fats, don't get enough protein, and suffer from nutritional deficiencies that increase their hunger level. Also, vegetarians who consume dairy products sometimes eat too much high-fat dairy, like cheese or full-fat yogurt, which drives up their saturated fat and calorie intake. Vegans, on the other hand, because they may have more difficulty finding a variety of protein-rich foods, can have a harder time maintaining balance in their diets. When that's the case, they too may end up overeating carbs and fats. There are a lot of ways to overeat, and it doesn't always involve consumption of animal foods.

RJ: Is soy bad for men?
EN: You mean does it make men grow breasts?

RJ: Yes! That's what I heard.
EN: No. It doesn't turn men into women. Soy contains something called isoflavones, also known as phytoestrogens. Phytoestrogens mimic the female hormone estrogen, although their estrogen-like activity is weak. So soy doesn't make men develop feminine characteristics, but it remains uncertain how phyto-

estrogens affect the growth of tumors related to breast cancer and diseases of the thyroid gland. It's important to note that soy has many health benefits. For example, when substituted for meats that contain saturated fats, soy has been shown to help reduce cholesterol levels. It's also rich in calcium and is useful in the prevention of osteoporosis. In certain cancers it has an anticarcinogenic effect, and it may help relieve menopausal symptoms too. The bottom line? If you have a history of breast cancer in your family or thyroid disease, you need to be careful and limit or avoid soy intake.

RJ: What's the deal with cheese? Does it clog up your body?

EN: All dairy products, except those that are nonfat, contain saturated fat, which may contribute to elevated cholesterol levels and increases the risk of heart disease. Dairy products also produce an insoluble residue in the lining of the intestines, which can be problematic for people with digestive issues like irritable bowel syndrome or inflammatory bowel disease. However, if you are able to digest dairy products without any reaction or difficulty, low-fat and nonfat versions are a great way to increase your protein and calcium intake.

RJ: I hear a lot of people complaining about lactose intolerance. Is that real?

EN: Yes, it's very real. People with lactose intolerance don't secrete enough of the digestive enzyme known as lactase, which breaks down a carbohydrate in milk called lactose.

Without enough lactase enzymes to digest them, dairy products can leave lactose-intolerant people with abdominal pain, gas, bloating, and possibly diarrhea. If you have a lactose intolerance and dairy foods are really important to you, you can use a digestive enzyme supplement prior to drinking milk or eating something like cheese or ice cream. Some people who have had gastric bypass surgery may temporarily develop lactose intolerance.

RJ: *I think I may have had it before, but after my surgery it got better.*

EN: That's unusual, but it may have to do with the amount of dairy you consume. Since your surgery, you're probably consuming smaller amounts of dairy products in one sitting, and smaller quantities are easier for the body to digest so there are fewer or less-intense side effects.

RJ: *Talk to me about vitamins. When you're trying to lose weight, do you need to take vitamins? I've also heard that vitamins can make you hungry.*

EN: There's no truth to the idea that vitamins make you hungry—unless you're substituting them for food. Of course, food is the best source of most vital nutrients, but as a backup plan, taking a multivitamin is helpful, to ensure that you get enough crucial micronutrients such as B vitamins, iron, zinc, magnesium, and calcium (especially important for post–gastric bypass patients). Antioxidant formulas are also useful for boosting immunity, promoting antiaging effects, and ensuring healthy energy levels. My favorite is Garden of Life's Perfect Food.

Also essential for good health are the omega-3 and -6 fatty acids found in fish and flaxseed oil. It's a good idea to regularly incorporate these foods into your diet, but if you don't, you might consider taking a supplement. Omega fatty acids are associated with a number of benefits including reduction in triglyceride levels, which is important for heart health. They also have natural anti-inflammatory power, help promote healthy digestive function, are excellent for arthritic pain, keep the skin and hair healthy, and help improve mood and mild symptoms of depression.

RJ: I take multi, iron, and B vitamins, which were recommended to me because after a gastric bypass you don't absorb as many nutrients. But the other day I saw this guy taking about twenty-three pills with his breakfast. I'm like, dude . . .

EN: That sounds like too much of a good thing. You definitely can overdo it with supplements, and some, such as iron, even have harmful toxic effects.

Blackened Pork Tenderloin

There is pork, and then there is *pork*. One has a lot of calories, the other is actually pretty lean. Tenderloin cuts have less fat than other cuts of meat (this goes for beef too), but what this dish lacks in fat it makes up in flavor from a spice rub.

Serves 4

Have on hand:
baking sheet
aluminum foil
cast-iron pan

1½ pounds pork tenderloin
1 tablespoon paprika
½ teaspoon kosher salt (optional)
1 teaspoon garlic powder
½ teaspoon cayenne
1 teaspoon ground black pepper
1 teaspoon ground white pepper
½ teaspoon dried thyme
1 cup fat-free chicken broth
8 oz no-salt-added tomato sauce

Preheat oven to 350°F. Line a baking sheet with aluminum foil; set aside.

Remove any silver skin left on tenderloin. Rinse under cold water and pat dry with paper towels. Thoroughly combine all seasonings (including salt if sodium is not an issue for you) and rub into pork. Allow pork to sit for 15 minutes for seasonings to cure. Pat in any remaining rub.

Heat a cast-iron pan over high heat until smoking hot. Sear pork on all sides until blackened and crusty. Remove from heat, transfer tenderloin to baking sheet, and roast in preheated oven for 10 to 15 minutes, or until internal temperature of pork reads 140°F.

Remove and let rest 10 minutes (internal temperature of pork will continue to rise to 145°F).

As pork rests, return pan to medium heat. Add broth to pan slowly (and carefully, as it will start to splatter). Scrape up browned bits in bottom of pan with a wooden spoon. Stir tomato sauce into pan and bring to a boil. Reduce heat to simmer for 5 to 10 minutes or until sauce has thickened.

Thinly slice pork diagonally and serve with pan sauce.

Per serving: *243 calories, 6 g fat (22.5% calories from fat), 40 g protein, 7 g carbohydrate, 2 g dietary fiber, 111 mg cholesterol, 228 mg sodium.*

Orange Zest Angel Food Cake with Blackberries

Angel food cake is very low in calories. This recipe calls for a mix, but you can also substitute a store-bought angel food cake and just prepare the topping.

Serves 12

<u>Have on hand</u>:
two 9-inch loaf pans
fine grater
juicer
small bowl
electric mixer
serrated knife

1 large orange
6 cups fresh or frozen blackberries
½ cup honey, divided
1 box angel food cake mix (such as Betty Crocker)
1 teaspoon orange extract, divided
3 cups nonfat plain yogurt
fresh mint sprigs, for garnish

Preheat oven to 350°F. Move oven rack to middle position. Have ready two 9-inch loaf pans, but do not grease.

Using a fine grater, remove zest from orange, then juice the zested orange. (One large orange yields approximately 1 tablespoon of zest and ¾ cup of juice.) Set aside.

In a small bowl, combine berries, ¼ cup honey, 1 teaspoon zest, and ¼ cup orange juice. Lightly toss to combine and let berries sit covered in refrigerator until ready to serve.

In a large mixing bowl, combine cake mix, remaining orange juice plus enough water to equal 1¼ cups, remaining orange zest, and ¾ teaspoon orange extract. Beat on low speed for 1 minute. Scrape down sides of bowl, then beat on medium speed for 1 minute more. Divide between the two ungreased loaf pans and bake for 35 to 45 minutes or until dark golden brown and cracked on the top. Do not underbake. Rest each loaf pan on its side until the cakes have completely cooled.

To make the topping, in a small bowl stir together yogurt, remaining ¼ cup honey, and remaining ¼ teaspoon orange extract.

To serve, run a knife around the edges of the loaf pans and remove cakes. Use a serrated knife to slice angel cake loafs into

¾-inch slices. For each serving, place 1 slice of cake on a chilled dessert plate. Top with ¼ cup berries, a little berry juice, and 2 tablespoons yogurt topping. Repeat with another layer and garnish with a sprig of mint. Store any unused cake tightly covered.

Per serving: 258 calories, trace fat (1.3% calories from fat), 7 g protein, 59 g carbohydrate, 4 g dietary fiber, 1 mg cholesterol, 364 mg sodium.

CHAPTER SIX

When and What to Eat

I want to talk more about the idea that you should eat when you're hungry. Having been a chronic meal skipper and someone who fought to ignore his hunger for so many years, answering the call of hunger was a big adjustment for me. (I should say answering the call of *mild* hunger, because, as I've noted, I would usually wait until I had to answer the insistent call of severe hunger.) But then came my diabetes diagnosis, and my former way of living had to go. To ensure that my blood sugar doesn't reach any treacherous highs or lows, I never go more than three or four hours without eating something. I eat several mini-meals a day, and because each "meal" (some of them are actually snacks) is small, I can pretty much predict that I'll be hungry again in a few hours.

Holding to this kind of schedule can be something of a challenge when I'm in a recording studio. The way musicians eat when they're making records is usually pretty terrible. For one thing, when you're in a studio you're working long hours, and you're in what is essentially a closed box. There's a computer screen, a panel of instruments, and a bunch of guitars and other musical accoutrements. And you're hanging out. For hours. And hours. You're barely conscious of time, and you're barely conscious of anything having to do with your body because you're in this euphoric state of making music. What happens, then, is that you go a very long time without eating. That might sound like a good thing, but eventually you have to acknowledge your growling stomach—you're famished. At this point you just want to make the hunger go away, and you don't particularly care if you do it in a nutritious or low-calorie way. It's like when you're a kid, it's summertime, and you're outside playing until nine o'clock at night, and you don't think about eating at all till you get home, at which point you gorge. As a kid, the most you have to deal with is your mom telling you to get out of the refrigerator. As an adult, you have to deal with the fact that your ravenous hunger led you to order up some burgers or pizza and beer, or some such stuff, none of which could be more fattening.

Sometimes if you are working at a high-end recording studio, they'll supply food. These setups of sandwiches and sweets are often a little better for you, but not much. These days I have a different solution, at least when I'm working in my own studio and I'm the producer in charge. First of all, I have a little refrigerator and a few shelves for food in my studio, and I stock the place with some healthy options. They're not perfect—I've got bags of those baked, fake Cheetos, which kind of taste like wood, and some diet sodas, along with things that are more nutritious like TLC and Lärabars—but they are there to tide me (and everyone else) over so I don't end up bingeing later.

The other thing I do is hire a caterer or chef to come in and make us healthy meals. No more ordering up greasy ribs and Chinese food. While making *Randy Jackson's Music Club, Volume 1*, which along with Paula, Elliott Yamin, and Katherine McPhee features Mariah Carey, Joss Stone, and Bebe Winans, among others, we had great meals of stir-fried vegetables and chicken, salads and lean slices of beef tenderloin.

I'm not telling you all this to get you to go out and hire a chef; I know that I'm in a privileged position to be able to have someone cook for me. What I'm trying to say is that if you plan for the situation you're going to be in, you can have a much better outcome. This might be as simple as bringing your lunch to work so that you don't end up eating fast food with your colleagues, who think nothing of chowing down on cheeseburgers every day. It might mean bringing along some chicken breasts to a family barbecue so that your only choice isn't fatty BBQ ribs. Maybe it means bringing along some fruit to business meetings that you know are going to go on for a long time.

This is especially important if you're going to be doing something that takes you away from your regular schedule. Say to yourself, "Look, we're going to be doing this for the next two months; let's not kill ourselves in the process. Let's make sure there are healthy snacks and meals available." That way you have a choice. You can sit back and let circumstances get the best of you (for me this would be going back to my old practice of waiting until I was famished, then speed-dialing the pizza place down the street) or you can take control of the situation by bringing food or, if you're going to be eating out or ordering in, gathering up the menus of all the places around you and finding out which restaurants have low-calorie options.

Eat When You Need To

A big part of planning ahead is making sure that you don't let vast expanses of time slip away without eating. That's the best way I know to set yourself up for some mad, crazy bingeing later on. Eating regularly, several times a day, is an approach that benefits everyone, diabetes or no diabetes. This doesn't mean you should eat when you're not hungry. If you're not experiencing physical signs of hunger (the first stomach rumblings, energy beginning to plummet), there's no reason to take in calories you don't need. You might not need that midmorning snack. Who knows? If you can go without a little something in the afternoon and not end up ravenous by dinnertime, then great. That works for you. I'm a firm believer in taking a theory and testing it out to find what's best for you as an individual.

Erin calls it following your "internal compass." If you have a light meal, you might be hungry in two hours. If you have a heavier meal, it might be four or five hours until you feel hungry again. What's most important—and I know I've said this a lot, but I think it's critical—is to be tuned in to your hunger level and to eat accordingly. If you have the sensation of hunger, have something that is satisfying—then stop when you feel satisfied or full (don't forget that part).

The exception to eating only when you feel hunger is breakfast. A lot of people aren't hungry when they first wake up in the morning. In the old days when I was skipping both breakfast and lunch, I never felt hungry first thing. But now I eat breakfast no matter what, and for a couple of different reasons. One of them is that if I don't, I'll eventually make up the calories—and then some. I know I can pass up breakfast and not feel incredibly hungry and that I can even make it through lunch without a drop of food. But I also know that later in the day, when my stamina takes a serious nosedive, I won't be able to stuff my face fast enough.

Even if you don't make it all the way to dinner like I used to, skipping breakfast is likely to trip you up in some way. And it makes sense if you think about it. When you get up in the morning, presuming you sleep the average seven or eight hours a night, the last time you ate was probably twelve or fourteen hours earlier. That's a long time to go without food. No wonder those coffee carts come around offices midmorning. They know there are going to be breakfast skippers trolling for a pastry fix. It's good business for them, but when you're trying to eat more healthfully, it's a bad situation for you.

There's also a physiological reason to eat every few hours. Eating gets your internal motor (i.e., your metabolism, the rate at which you burn calories) running so you actually burn more calories when you eat than when you don't eat. If you go several hours without food, your body starts to conserve energy, which means that it's not going to burn as many calories as it would if you gave it a little nudge by way of a piece of toast with peanut butter or a bowl of cereal. So by not eating first thing in the morning, you actually do yourself a disservice.

I don't want to overstate the metabolism thing. Having breakfast isn't going to suddenly turn your body into a pumped-up, calorie-burning machine. That skinny guy down the street who can eat twelve grilled cheese sandwiches without gaining an ounce is still going to burn more calories than you. But eating in the morning—and at intervals throughout the day—will bump up your calorie burning a little and, hey, every calorie counts.

Eating breakfast doesn't mean you have to sit down to a full meal. At least have something, though, even if it's just a banana or a few bites of yogurt or a handful of almonds. You've probably heard all that breakfast hype out there, but in this case the hype is true: it really does get you going on the right foot, by improving concentration and stamina. Plus, people who eat breakfast actually do tend to be healthier and thinner too.

The key thing to remember about eating more often is that it doesn't mean having a three-course meal six times a day. Eat often, but eat *small* amounts. You might, for instance, have a salad for lunch but save the apple and crackers you'd usually eat with it for midafternoon. Breakfast might be a bowl of cereal, and for a midmorning snack, you might have some yogurt. I've found that it helps me be more inclined to listen to my fullness signals if I know that I'm going to be able to eat again a few hours later.

As I said, eating more often requires planning, something that didn't come naturally to me. I was never the guy who took a brown bag to work. I still don't, but I now know the healthy places I can order from near my office, and I'll put an energy bar, peach, or apple in my pocket if I know I'm going to be in meetings or at an *Idol* taping for several hours. Especially in the early part of the *Idol* season, we put in long hours and we spend three, often four, days a week shooting. I always make sure there is something, and preferably something nutritious and fairly low cal, available. That's the other part of this. Eating more frequently can help you cut calories, but not if you're eating junk. It's easier to resist junk food, though, if you're not out-of-control hungry.

Eating several times a day can also take some mental fine-tuning. If you've struggled with your weight for a long time, the idea of eating frequently might freak you out. But get over it. Being able to withstand hunger is not a badge of honor, because inevitably you're going to compensate for those feelings of deprivation. Stoicism now will only lead to disorderly conduct later.

The Write Stuff: How Keeping a Food Journal Can Help

Quick—do you know what you ate so far today? A few years ago I probably couldn't have told you myself. Like a lot of people, I ate unconsciously. If you've ever woken up to the fact that you've gained ten pounds but not known where it came from, then you probably eat unconsciously too. Don't blame it on a slow metabolism. Or at least not until you take a look at what you're *really* eating.

At this point, it's become sort of a diet cliché: keep a food journal. But that's because it really works. There's no better way to check up on yourself. It's a great way to get connected to your feelings of hunger and fullness and to find out what foods satisfy you the most. I started keeping a food journal when I was first diagnosed with diabetes because I honestly didn't think I was doing that badly. I wanted to see what was going on. Well, it turns out I wasn't doing as well as I thought, and because it was all there in black and white, I couldn't really deny it. Besides simply documenting what I was eating (too much, not such good stuff), the journal shed some light on what times of day and in what situations I was most vulnerable to overeating. It was also a valuable tool for looking at when I *didn't* overeat. What was it about those times that allowed me to be satisfied with less? Was it the particular foods I was eating? Or was it because I was eating quietly and paying attention to my food rather than eating and doing a million things at once? These are just some of the questions that chronicling my food life helped me to answer.

There are a lot of different ways to keep a food journal, but Erin suggests using a three-step approach that lets you focus on one aspect of eating at a time. Here's how to go about it.

Step One

What you're going to do first is use your journal as Appetite Awareness 101. Your mission is to document how hungry you feel before you eat and how full you feel when you stop. Write down everything you eat, and I mean everything: not just your meals, but all the little bites you have here and there. Incidental eating. I'm talking about the double latte you grabbed on the way to work. The packet of pretzels you pulled from the vending machine. The handful of crackers you grabbed while you were cooking dinner. The half a sandwich your daughter left on her plate and you didn't want to let go to waste. The granola bar you ate in the car while driving to an appointment.

Don't focus on how much of the food you ate or whether it was junky or nutritious. Just write down the feelings of hunger (or lack of them) that led up to your putting food in your mouth, be it at a meal or otherwise. Did you eat because the food was there or because your rumbling stomach told you to? Then note the flip side: how full were you when you put that last crumb of cookie in your mouth? Stuffed or just comfortable? Use the Hunger and Satiety Scale on page 101 to help you. Keeping your journal with you at all times will help you keep more accurate entries, but I can also see where you might not want to lug a book around. If that's the case, record everything on small pieces of paper throughout the day, then transfer the info into your journal later.

Step Two

Hopefully, after a couple of weeks of following step one, you'll be more conscious of when you're truly hungry and adequately full. Now you're going to work on *how* full the foods you're eating make you feel. You know how they always say that when you eat Chinese food you're hungry an hour later? This is to see whether that kind of thing is true.

Your assignment this time around is to write down the effects of the different types of foods you're eating. For instance, I generally feel fuller faster and longer if I have something like chicken satay for lunch than if I have a simple green salad. That's likely for two reasons: because protein is known to trigger satiety quickly, and because the peanut sauce that comes with chicken satay provides the fat that will keep me full for a fairly long while after I'm done (fat takes longer to digest than protein or carbs).

I'm a believer in the idea that you've got to find the foods that work for you, and this is one way to do it. It's all part of really paying attention to what's going on in your body so that you make better choices. Besides writing down how satisfying different foods are, also write down how they make you feel. If you feel pretty nauseated after eating a box of cookies, write it down. Don't sweep this stuff under the rug! You're going to be more likely to change this particular habit if you're able to weigh the fact that cookies taste good against the fact that the way you overeat them makes you feel sick. Keep it real!

Step Three

Here comes the hard part: portion sizes. When you're used to eating a big platter of food, scaling down is difficult, and I say this even as a man who had a big incentive—a band around my stomach—to do so. Old habits die hard. But they don't die at all unless you start looking at them, so use your journal as a way to get a read on exactly how much you're eating. Again, you don't have to measure your food, but guesstimate it, then compare it to what's considered a moderate serving size (see page 128).

What you should be looking at, too, is the balance of your portions throughout the day. It might not be so bad to have two or three servings of rice at lunch, but not if you're also having two or three servings at dinner. This is the time to check it out and see where you can live with cutting back.

It bears repeating that keeping a food journal, even if it's just for a few weeks, can be incredibly helpful. I kept mine for a couple of years. No one was going to check up on how I was eating; I had to do it myself, and the journal provided a good way to keep myself honest and prevent backsliding. When I did slip up, the act of writing it down helped me think about why and whether I got anything out of it. Yeah, that coffee cake was good, but was it worth it? Sometimes the answer was yes, but more often the answer was just plain no.

Look at Portion Sizes, Not Calories

In the body-conscious town of Hollywood, there are people who can tell you the exact number of calories in everything from a pea to a piece of Wolfgang Puck pizza. They're like walking food databases. I gave up counting calories a long time ago. That doesn't mean I can't look at most foods and tell you whether or not they're fattening (at least when you eat them in large and sometimes even moderate amounts). I became very familiar with calorie counts during all those years of dieting.

I think it's a good idea to look at package labels and nutrition information whenever you can so you know how many calories are in the foods you typically eat. (The calorie counts of the popular fast-food meals on page 32, for instance, might surprise you.) That said, counting calories all day long can make you crazy. The better way to ensure that you don't take in too many calories is—that's right—to listen to your body and moderate your portion sizes.

Ultimately, the arbiter of how much you eat at any sitting will be your body's satiety signals. Stop when you feel the first stirrings of fullness—that's the rule. But you'll be a lot less likely to eat beyond that point if you don't already have a huge serving on your plate. That's where moderate portion sizes come in.

I never thought I'd hear myself say this, but I love in-flight airplane meals. Well, not the meals themselves, really (I think we can agree that they're usually not fine dining), but the way they're laid out and the little sectioned plates they come on. You've got your chicken, beef, or pasta in a section about the size of your palm; your little vegetable on the side; a fist-sized salad with just about a tablespoon of dressing; one roll; a small pat of butter; and a piece of cake about half the size of a deck of cards. It's perfect! Not too much, not too little. Moderate.

This is the visual I have in my head when I eat a meal. At

home it's easy. I just take care to dish myself out portions that jibe with the airline meal. At restaurants, of course, it's harder. In fact, most restaurant portions (including, and perhaps especially, fast-food portions) are way too big. Have you seen the size of some of those burgers? Dude! There's enough for three people. Still, even if I'm served a plate of pasta that could feed a small country, I keep that airline plate in my mind's eye and try not to eat past it.

There are a couple of other visual cues that might help you keep your portions down to a reasonable size. Here are three:

Meat, chicken, fish = palm of your hand
Rice, noodles, cereal, and other grains = tennis ball
Cheeses = one thumb

Portion sizes of fruits and vegetables are of less concern, unless you're eating vegetables cooked in butter or oil (in that case, keep it to half a tennis ball). Dessert? Think back to the cake on the airline meal plate: about half the size of a deck of cards. And while we're on the subject, let's talk more about sweets and some of the other foods it's hard to live without.

Occasionally Give In to Your Cravings

One thing I love to do is sit outside at a corner café where I can watch the traffic go by and listen to what kind of music people are rocking out to in their cars. Sometimes it's pure bubblegum—catchy, mushy, insubstantial, but pleasurable. Does that person live on a steady diet of bubblegum or is he just indulging a bit? Could be either. Even if you live on a lofty diet of Coltrane and Miles, sometimes you've just got to hear something sweet and easy.

Likewise when it comes to food. No matter how healthfully you're trying to eat, there are going to be times when you want a piece of cake or pie or some other food that has a ton of calories. Whenever I was on a diet, this is what I would call the "cheat moment." But is it really cheating? To my revised way of thinking, no. According to the diet mentality, you are either all good or all bad. But what I realized is that if you're eating healthfully most of the time, there is nothing wrong with now and then eating something that's not particularly healthy, just because you like it. And it *does* matter what you call it. The word *cheating* is negative. If you have that word in your head, you're going to feel guilty about doing something that might even help you stay on the straight and narrow.

The problem with placing strict limits on the kinds of foods you can eat is that when you slip up—and who doesn't on occasion?—it makes you feel like a complete failure. I threw in the towel on many a diet because I fell off the so-called wagon. It seemed that if I couldn't follow *all* the rules, I shouldn't follow *any* of the rules. Next thing you know, I'd be "cheating" on that diet on a full-time basis.

A lot of what drives the choices we make about eating is how we *think* about eating. That's why it's so important to give yourself a break. It's not cheating to allow yourself something sinful once in a while, and, as I said before, it can even help.

Artificial Sweeteners: Yes or No?

Sometimes I have a diet root beer. Sometimes I put an artificial sweetener in my coffee or ice tea. I'll have a Diet Coke now and then too. The FDA thinks artificial sweeteners are safe, but some scientists aren't so sure, so in my mind the jury is still out. To be honest, I don't think they're the best thing for you. Yet while I'm trying to eat as many natural foods as I can these days, once in a while I need a serious hit of sweetness without the spike in blood sugar I'd get from real sugar. That's when a diet root beer comes in real handy.

But I am working to cut back on sugar substitutes for a couple of reasons. One is that the sweetness is so intense (I think they taste even sweeter than sugar) that it always makes me crave salt. I've got that sweet-salty thing going on. I guess a lot of people do. There's a reason why soft drinks and pizza, milkshakes and fries, movie popcorn and candy go together like Lennon and McCartney (that's the Beatles, for you kids out there). So by keeping artificial sweeteners to a minimum, I'm also hoping to keep my desire for salty foods like chips from cropping up.

As I talk about on page 130, there's also something to the idea that when you have a fake anything, you're not going to be truly satisfied. Here's Erin's take on it: "It's like your taste buds are telling your body, 'sugar is on the way' but then nothing, meaning no calories, arrives," she says. In other words, your body is gypped! That's got to make you feel unsatisfied and get you longing for more food. So are artificial sweeteners going to help you consume fewer calories in the end? Maybe, but be aware of what you're consuming so that you don't go looking for the missing calories elsewhere.

Have the bowl of ice cream you're craving and you're not going to turn into that angry person so pissed off about deprivation that you head to Fosters Freeze for a three-scoop sundae and a bucket of fries for good measure.

Here's the other thing: I really think that, in most cases, if you are craving a doughnut, you should have a doughnut. Half a doughnut, but a doughnut. If you really want a piece of apple pie, you should have a small slice of apple pie. Not every day and maybe not in the portion sizes you used to have—have that airline-sized dessert instead—but have the real thing. If you try to fake out your body with a substitute, you're not going to be satisfied. Chances are, you're going to go looking for something else. I know that if I'm craving something, I can have a thousand rice cakes but I'm still going to want it. Sometimes you've just got to have something *good*.

Here's another example. Say your significant other brings home some cupcakes left over from a party at work. You're trying to lose weight. Cupcakes are off your list. Yet there they are, occupying counter space in your kitchen and, worse, occupying your mind. You can hardly pay attention to the phone conversation you're having because you want them so bad. So you go to the freezer and have a diet fudge pop. That didn't satisfy you, so now you have a few crackers. Nope. Now a banana. Maybe you ate healthier foods, but you also ate twice the calories of one little cupcake in your effort to be "good." If you had the cupcake or, better yet, half of it, it would have been over. You could have just gotten on with your life and returned to normal, healthy eating.

I'm not saying that you should never defer to lower calorie substitutes. They can really work. I'm also not saying that you should give in to your cravings every day. What I'm getting at is that if you sometimes let yourself have a food you love, you're going to reduce the chances of either overcompensating by accident or completely falling apart and giving up on healthier habits.

So, like I said, on these occasions I let myself have the real thing but in smaller portions. I can't have the whole banana cream pie, but I can have a couple of bites. I can't have a big hunk of chocolate cake, but I can have a sliver. Let me reiterate: I'm a big fan of the "morsel diet." I eat slowly and savor each bite, and it seems to work. Disaster averted. Sometimes a square of chocolate is actually a better choice than a rice cake.

The Foods You Choose

Today I had a beautiful salad for lunch. It had all kinds of different greens, a little avocado, a little chicken, some shredded carrots, tomatoes, herbs, and a nice citrus dressing. Would I have had that for lunch a few years ago? No, but it's delicious to me now. My typical lunch used to be a cheeseburger, fries, and a milkshake or maybe fried chicken and a root beer or a big ol' plate of red beans and rice. But I've changed my outlook. I see the salad as really fresh, colorful, and, most important, health-ful. And I actually like it. A lot.

I used to know every bakery in town; now I know every bakery and natural foods market that sells juice-sweetened, whole grain cakes and cookies. Some of that healthy stuff can be pretty terrible—I'm the first to admit it. But I've done a lot of research and some healthy pastries are actually very tasty. So, sure, sometimes I might prefer a piece of real chocolate cake made in the traditional way with butter and sugar ga-lore. Or a real piece of peach pie. But on a more regular basis, I have found nutritious substitutes and made my peace with that.

How did I do it? There was no magic involved. It was really a combination of two things. The first thing is that I started to think about food differently. I am a recovering diabetic. I sim-ply can't have certain foods. Or let me put it another way: I can have anything I want, but I *choose* not to have certain foods. Because I know it's not going to end happily for me. It's not that I have stopped loving doughnuts or the kind of everything-in-the-pot gumbo my mom used to make. But I am married to my disease. I want to make choices that make me feel good both physically and emotionally. So although I have free will, I use it to do the right thing. That's in my best interest.

If you don't have diabetes, you might not feel like you have an imperative to learn to love healthier foods. But, be-lieve me, you do. Being overweight puts you on the path to diabetes, heart disease, and a host of other problems. The lat-est thing I read is that researchers now believe that obesity increases your risk of cancer. There are a lot of bad things about being fat, and maybe you're focused on the fact that you don't like the way you look. That's a good reason to change, but my experience has been that health is the bigger motivator. If you think of being overweight as a disease, just like an alcoholic or a drug addict thinks of his affliction as a disease, you're going to have an easier time setting parameters for yourself.

Here is something else that's relevant: you can get used to just about anything. You know, it's like that pop song you hear on the radio and hate because it's, well, so poppy, but then you keep hearing it in your head and you start liking it. Pretty soon you're moving around on the dial trying to find it. (I'm not saying Jason got so used to interviews that he started seeking them out, but who knows?! Maybe he did.) It can take several weeks, but if you begin eating healthier foods, you will start to get used to them and even to like them. If you have ever changed from whole milk to low-fat milk, you know what I mean. The low fat tastes watery at first, but after a while the whole milk tastes too rich. It can be the same with other foods. When you're used to low-sugar cereals, the sugary ones start to taste over-the-top sweet. Whole wheat bread begins to taste nutty and flavor-rich, white bread bland and mundane. You're not going to like everything and sometimes, like I noted earlier, nothing but the real thing will do. But on an everyday basis, you can adapt to changes if you give it time.

So what, specifically, should you eat? What I love to eat and what you love to eat might be two completely different things. That's another of the many reasons I believe that diets can fail you: they often expect everyone to be happy eating the same food and don't bear in mind cultural or individual differences. So I'm not going to tell you exactly what you *should* eat. What I'm going to do instead is offer some ideas that might work for you.

One of the hardest things about eating healthfully is figuring out what to have at any given time of the day. The list of meal and snack suggestions on the upcoming pages is here to help you when you're stuck for ideas and to show you what a healthy eating plan looks like. You're welcome to follow the suggestions to the letter, mix them up, or pick and choose as you see fit. Whatever suits you. Just know that they are all healthy, moderate-calorie recommendations, and that they can help you put all the strategies I've talked about in this chapter, and throughout the book, into play.

Two Weeks' Worth of Good Eats

If you've been on and off a million diets, the structure of the fourteen-day meal plan below might look familiar. But there's a difference, the biggest one being that it's more free-form. There are very few specific serving sizes—this is so *you* can determine how much you need to be eating. As Erin, who developed this plan, says, one daily calorie count does not fit all: the number of calories I need as a 225-pound man are much greater than the calorie needs of someone tiny like my friend Paula Abdul. But beyond that, the most critical determinant of how much you should eat is your own level of hunger and satiety. You might keep in mind the moderate portion sizes I discussed on page 128 so you'll know about how much to start out with. Then listen to your body: eat only when you're truly physically hungry, and stop when you feel the first sensations of fullness.

That's what's really going to help you cut back on calories. If it's not working and you're not losing weight over time (remember, this isn't drastic calorie cutting so you have to be patient), then you know you have to make a more conscious effort to cut a few more calories here and there. Make small changes so that you can live with them.

While these menus provide you with fourteen different full-day plans, again, feel free to mix up the breakfasts, lunches, and dinners or to combine them with your own choices. (The dishes in bold type refer to recipes in this book.) However you plan out your day, though, include a good mix of protein, fat, and carbohydrates, and try to eat a variety of different foods. Each food brings its own set of vitamins, minerals, and disease-fighting phytochemicals to the table, so the more variety in your diet the better.

Most of all, choose the meals that will give you pleasure. Remember, you're not dieting anymore. You want to eat this way for life, and the only way you're going to be able to do that is if you find the happy medium between foods that make you happy and foods that make you healthy.

	Monday Day 1	**Tuesday** Day 2	**Wednesday** Day 3
BREAK-FAST	• Fiber-rich cereal (at least 4 grams of fiber per serving), such as: oatmeal, Müeslix, Kashi cereal, raisin bran, Fiber One, All-Bran, Cracklin' Oat Bran, Grape-Nuts • 1 cup 1% or nonfat milk or calcium-fortified soy milk • 1 banana or apple	• Egg or egg white omelet with diced vegetables (e.g., tomatoes, bell peppers, onions, spinach, mush-rooms, sun-dried tomatoes) and shredded low-fat cheese • Whole-wheat toast	• Granola yogurt parfait made with low-fat granola, plain or flavored non- or low-fat yogurt, and a cup of blueberries
LUNCH	• Shrimp with dill and lemon • Angel hair pasta • Side salad	• Tuna sandwich on whole-wheat bread • Fruit salad or baked chips	• Turkey wrap with whole-wheat tortilla, avocado, toma-toes, spinach, and hummus spread • **Oatmeal apple spice cookie**
DINNER	• Teriyaki chicken or tofu • Quinoa • Asparagus • **Chewy pecan cran-berry bar**	• **Turkey meat loaf with tomato gravy** • Wild rice and grilled veg-etables	• **Blackened pork tender-loin** • Green salad or tomato basil soup • Small fruit tart

	Thursday Day 4	**Friday** Day 5	**Saturday** Day 6
BREAK-FAST	• Nutrition bar, such as Clif bar, Lunabar, Lärabar, granola bar, Genisoy • 1 cup of 1% or nonfat milk or calcium-fortified soy milk	• English muffin with cottage cheese (optional: topped with honey and cinnamon) • 1 cup of chopped cantaloupe	• Pancakes made from whole-wheat mix with blueberries or favorite fruit, chopped, thrown into the batter (eat plain or top with additional chopped fruit and 2 tablespoons low-fat vanilla yogurt)
LUNCH	• Tofu or chicken stir-fry with vegetables and noodles • Low-fat rice pudding	• Grilled vegetable and chicken quesadilla with pico de gallo and black beans • Optional: spoonful of guacamole or sour cream	• Turkey or vegetarian chili • Whole grain roll • Lemon bar
DINNER	• **Chicken étouffée** • Salad • **Low-fat sweet potato pie with pecan crust**	• Grilled salmon • Vegetable couscous • Sauteed green beans • Mango sorbet	• **Double-dipped buttermilk oven-fried chicken** • Brown rice • Brussels sprouts sautéed with olive oil and garlic

	Day 7	Day 8	Day 9
BREAK-FAST	• Scrambled eggs or egg whites • Turkey sausage or vegetarian breakfast links • Rosemary potatoes • 1 cup straw-berries	• Smoothie made with: 1 cup juice, 1% or nonfat milk, or calcium-fortified soy milk; ½ cup frozen ber-ries; 1 table-spoon wheat germ; and, for protein, 6 oz low-fat or nonfat flavored yogurt, 3 oz tofu or protein powder or **big berry burst**	• Oatmeal made with long-cooking oats cooked in calcium-fortified soy milk or 1% or nonfat milk, topped with 1 cup chopped apples and blueberries, and 1 to 2 tablespoons chopped wal-nuts
LUNCH	• Vegetable and cheese frittata • Whole grain toast • Fruit salad	• Smoked turkey on whole grain roll with avo-cado, lettuce, and tomato • Fruit salad or baked chips	• **Citrus and toasted al-mond salad** with grilled chicken breast • Whole grain pita
DINNER	• Tuna steak on whole grain bun with lettuce, tomatoes, and chopped veg-etable salad • **Orange zest angel food cake with black-berries**	• **Shrimp and sausage gumbo ya ya** • Grilled aspara-gus • Wild rice • Small piece of chocolate	• Grilled tuna • Garlic rice • Sautéed spinach • Mango and berry fruit salad

	Day 10	Day 11	Day 12
BREAK-FAST	• Hard-boiled egg(s) • Whole-wheat toast with 1 teaspoon butter or peanut butter • 1 cup mixed berries topped with a spoonful of low-fat yogurt and 1 teaspoon of honey	• Bagel with 1 tablespoon peanut butter or almond butter • 1 cup low-fat or nonfat milk or calcium-fortified soy milk • Source of protein: eggs or turkey sausage	• Cream of wheat sweetened with applesauce and cinnamon, topped with chopped hard-boiled egg
LUNCH	• Barbecued chicken or tofu pizza with broccoli, onions, and zucchini • Small green salad	• Egg salad sandwich on whole-wheat baguette with low-fat mayonnaise • Fruit salad	• Tuna and avocado wrap on whole-wheat tortilla • Small green salad with balsamic vinaigrette dressing
DINNER	• Halibut with olive oil, garlic, and dill • Tomato basil soup • Whole grain roll • **Perfect peach cobbler**	• **Quick-cooking creole-style sea bass** • **NOLA red beans and rice**	• **Spaghetti squash with spicy turkey meatballs in tomato sauce** • Chopped grilled vegetable salad

	Day 13	Day 14
BREAK-FAST	• High-fiber waffle (frozen or from mix), topped with 1 cup sliced strawberries, 1 tablespoon organic maple syrup, and 2 teaspoons butter or butter alternative • 1 cup 1% or nonfat milk or calcium-fortified soy milk or 2 scrambled eggs	• Breakfast burrito made with eggs or egg whites, pinto or black beans, 2 tablespoons shredded cheese, and 1/8 avocado wrapped in a high-fiber tortilla
LUNCH	• Tofu or shrimp kabobs with grilled eggplant and bell peppers • Orzo salad • Oatmeal raisin cookie	• **Hoppin' John soup** • Seeded whole grain roll • Spinach salad with dried cranberries, pine nuts, and tomatoes
DINNER	• Lasagna Rollups • Spicy southern collards • **Banana pudding pie**	• Tilapia fish tacos with corn tortillas, shredded cabbage, and salsa • Flaxseed tortilla chips with pico de gallo

Go Ahead—Eat Between Meals

One of the great things about touring with a rock band is that you get to travel all over Europe. I love it. I love playing France, Italy, Germany. I love London, Stockholm, Oslo. Traveling over there allows you to soak up entirely different ideas about living. One thing I learned while touring Europe is that most Europeans eat very differently than we do. For breakfast you've got juice, coffee, some toast or brioche with butter or an English muffin with jam. It's small, though. Not like our big American breakfast with an omelet filled with eighteen things.

The other thing is, they don't generally eat snacks. They tend to really luxuriate in their meals, taking their time and eating to a point where they can hold out for the several hours till their next sit-down. Americans don't really operate that way. We're more on the go; we don't hang out and eat two- or three-hour lunches. That type of lifestyle, combined with the demands of having diabetes and a surgically altered stomach, has made me an unapologetic snacker. I really depend on them to get me through the day and to keep me from overeating at meals.

There are two rules of thumb I try to stick to when it comes to snacks. One is to have a snack when I need it, not just because I've set a plan for myself to have two or three snacks a day. If I'm not hungry, I don't eat, and if I am hungry, I decide how much I'm going to eat based on fullness. What goes for meals goes for snacks too.

The other thing I try to do is always have something on hand. I mentioned earlier that I often bring along a protein bar or shake if I know I'm going to be locked up in the studio or in meetings for hours on end. That's just one option. "You might, for instance, keep a small bag of nuts or raisins in your desk as a safety net for low-energy emergencies," says Erin. "Throw a banana, orange, or tangerine—something that won't get smashed—in your purse or pocket before you leave for the day." Think ahead whenever you can and try to anticipate every possible scenario. If you know your kids are going to beg you to stop for fast food after soccer practice, bring along a yogurt to eat while you watch them play so that you're not hungry enough to give in to their pleas on the way home.

Snacks are only helpful when they're satisfying. A couple of carrot sticks aren't going to do it for me—but that's not to say they won't do it for you. A lot of it's individual. And it can be different on different days, depending on my mood. Some days I'm happy with just about anything; other days I have real strong cravings and it helps to placate them. Because, like I keep saying, if you really have a strong desire for something, you'll probably end up having it anyway. Better to have, say, a small piece of chocolate or a little chocolate pudding as your snack than to have some cheese and crackers and the candy on top of it. You end up with double the calories.

Erin has another suggestion about snack choices: when you can, choose a snack that contains a combination of protein, carbohydrates, and fat. A graham cracker with some peanut butter, for instance, or a piece of cheese with a cracker. "A snack doesn't have to have all three to be a good choice, but the combination of protein, fat, and carbs will make you feel fuller and keep you going longer than a snack made up of just one macronutrient," says Erin. Here's a list of healthy possibilities.

- Low or nonfat yogurt with low-fat granola, chopped fruit, berries, or nuts
- Cantaloupe with cottage cheese and a drizzle of honey
- Trail mix
- A cup of berries
- Low-fat rice pudding, chocolate pudding, or tapioca pudding

- Banana or apple slices spread with peanut butter
- Low-fat whole grain crackers with cottage cheese or a slice of cheese
- A slice of deli meat wrapped around a piece of avocado
- String cheese and pretzels
- Edamame (soy beans) with low-sodium soy sauce
- Hard-boiled egg with crackers or pita bread
- Tuna salad and crackers
- Oatmeal raisin cookie and 1 percent or nonfat milk or calcium-fortified soy milk
- A square of chocolate (preferably dark, which has anti-oxidants)
- Bagel or English muffin half spread with peanut or almond butter
- Half a sandwich or wrap made with turkey or soy meat, a slice of cheese, lettuce and tomato, and low-fat ranch dressing
- Protein bar such as Balance Bar, Clif Bar, PowerBar, Kashi, Luna bar, Lärabar, ExtendBar, or Genisoy
- One-quarter cup nuts (approximately twenty pieces): choose from walnuts, peanuts, almonds, cashews, or pistachios, then prepackage in ziplock bags and have them ready to go
- Vegetables, such as carrots, celery, cherry tomatoes, cucumbers, or peppers, and dip, such as low-fat cottage cheese, low-fat cream cheese, *tzatziki* (Greek yogurt-cucumber dip), or hummus

Citrus and Toasted Almond Salad

To make a complete meal, toss in 4 oz of grilled salmon or skinless chicken breast.

Serves 6

Have on hand:
Small and large bowls
baking sheet

FOR DRESSING

- ¼ cup fresh orange juice
- ¼ cup fresh lemon juice
- 1 teaspoon Dijon mustard
- 1 teaspoon grated ginger root
- 1½ tablespoons extra-virgin olive oil

FOR SALAD

- 2 pink grapefruits
- 2 oranges
- 8 cups baby spinach leaves
- 1 cup chopped red bell pepper
- ½ avocado, peeled and sliced (optional)
- ½ cup sliced almonds, toasted*
- ⅓ cup crumbled goat cheese (optional)

*To toast almonds, preheat oven to 350°F. Spread almonds evenly on a baking sheet and roast for 7 to 10 minutes, until fragrant and lightly golden. Stir once to ensure even browning.

Prepare dressing by whisking together orange juice, lemon juice, mustard, and ginger in a small bowl. Slowly whisk in olive oil. Set aside.

Remove peeling and pith from grapefruits and oranges. Cut sections into bite-size pieces. In a large bowl combine spinach, grapefruit and orange segments, and bell pepper.

Whisk dressing and measure out ¼ cup. Pour ¼ cup dressing over salad and gently toss. Divide dressed salad among 6 plates and garnish with sliced avocado, toasted almonds, and crumbled goat cheese. Serve remaining dressing on the side.

Per serving: 192 calories, 13 g fat (54.2% calories from fat), 5 g protein, 19 g carbohydrate, 4 g dietary fiber, 0 mg cholesterol, 45 mg sodium.

Turkey Meat Loaf with Tomato Gravy

To me, meat loaf is good comfort food. In this low-calorie version, the comfort comes without a side of guilt.

Serves 8

<u>Have on hand</u>:
9×13 inch baking dish
canola oil cooking spray
large nonstick skillet
large bowl
small saucepan

½ cup finely chopped onion

½ cup finely chopped celery

½ green bell pepper, finely chopped

2 teaspoons minced garlic

1 tablespoon Tabasco sauce

1½ teaspoons low-sodium soy sauce

6 tablespoons chili sauce, divided

2 egg whites, lightly beaten

⅓ cup evaporated skim milk

1 cup old-fashioned rolled oats

1¼ pounds ground turkey breast

FOR GRAVY

1 can (8 oz) tomato sauce

2 teaspoons balsamic vinegar

1 teaspoon soy sauce

Preheat oven to 350°F. Lightly spray a 9×13 inch baking dish with canola oil cooking spray.

Heat oil in a large nonstick skillet over medium-high heat. Sauté vegetables until soft, about 5 to 7 minutes. Add Tabasco, soy sauce, and 3 tablespoons chili sauce. Transfer to a large bowl to cool.

When vegetables have cooled, stir in egg whites, evaporated milk, and rolled oats. Add turkey and mix well with your hands (mixture will be very moist).

Form into a loaf and place in the prepared baking dish. Spread remaining chili sauce over top. Bake in middle of oven for 50 to 55 minutes, or until thermometer registers 170°F.

For gravy: Combine sauce ingredients in a small saucepan and warm until heated through.

Let meat loaf rest 5 minutes before slicing. Serve with warmed sauce.

Per serving: *158 calories, 3g fat (18.9% calories from fat), 19g protein, 13g carbohydrate, 2g dietary fiber, 40mg cholesterol, 452mg sodium.*

Chewy Pecan Cranberry Bars

In another life, I would have never considered anything with so many healthy ingredients—oats, pecans, cranberries, and yogurt—dessert. I guess I didn't know what I was missing!

Serves 16

Have on hand:
9×13 inch baking pan
canola oil cooking spray
medium and large mixing bowls
wire cooling rack

2½ cups quick-cooking oats
1 cup puffed rice cereal (such as Rice Krispies)
½ cup chopped pecans
½ cup dried cranberries
¾ cup packed brown sugar
2 egg whites, lightly beaten
½ cup honey

1 cup low-fat plain yogurt
2 tablespoons canola oil
1 teaspoon vanilla extract
1 cup flour
½ teaspoon kosher salt
1 teaspoon ground cinnamon

Preheat oven to 350°F. Lightly spray 9×13 inch baking pan with canola cooking spray. Set aside.

Combine oats, cereal, pecans, and cranberries in a medium bowl. Set aside.

Stir together sugar, beaten eggs, honey, yogurt, oil, and vanilla extract in a large mixing bowl. Sift together flour, salt, and cinnamon and stir into yogurt mixture.

Stir in oat mixture. Transfer to the prepared pan and spread evenly. Bake in preheated oven for 20 to 25 minutes, or until lightly browned. Cool completely on wire rack. Cut into 16 squares and store in airtight container.

Per serving: *204 calories, 5 g fat (22.9% calories from fat), 4 g protein, 36 g carbohydrate, 2 g dietary fiber, 1 mg cholesterol, 82 mg sodium.*

Big Berry Burst

This smoothie makes a great snack, breakfast drink, or post-workout revitalizer.

Serves 2

Have on hand:
blender

> **1½ cups frozen blackberries or mixed berries**
> **1 banana, cut in large chunks**
> **1 cup low-calorie cranberry juice**
> **3 tablespoons nonfat dry milk powder**
> **whey protein power (optional)**
> **ice, as needed**

Add all ingredients except ice to blender and whir on high speed until blended. Add enough ice to create smoothie. Pour into glasses and serve.

Per serving: *172 calories, 1 g fat (3.9% calories from fat), 4 g protein, 40 g carbohydrate, 7 g dietary fiber, 1 mg cholesterol, 40 mg sodium.*

CHAPTER SEVEN

Idol, Not Idle

I like to hold meetings at hotels. If I'm on a big project, like *Randy Jackson Presents America's Best Dance Crew,* and I've got to talk to journalists or chat up talent, I'll have them hang with me at one of LA's better spots. Many of these hotels have gyms, so you'll be sitting there talking and a stream of people in workout clothes will walk back and forth. And, you know, most of them are very thin.

But are they thin *because* they go to the gym? Aha! That is the sixty-four-thousand-dollar question. I think some people really do get thin by going to the gym regularly and working off the croissants. But many regular gym goers are also thin by nature, and a lot of people who are not so thin don't really feel comfortable going to a health club. When it comes to gyms, I'm a love 'em and leave 'em kind of guy. Over the years, I must have belonged to twenty gyms and have had more than a few trainers. It just doesn't work for me. If it works for you, that's great, especially if you belong to a gym that has a lot of options—like twenty varieties of cardio machines and a smorgasbord of exercise classes—to keep you from becoming bored. Sometimes having a trainer is an awesome way to get fit: you can't slack off when someone is standing there watching you (and you're paying him for it too!). But that said, you don't need a trainer or a gym membership to get fit.

For me, working out had to be very simple. That's why I love walking. You can do it anywhere, anytime, alone or with someone. In my book it's the answer to the imperative "just get moving." Now I exercise every day. That's proof that you don't have to have fancy equipment or someone calling you on the carpet to be an active person.

It's possible that I don't like the gym because I spent so much time working out in one when I was young and training for football and other sports. After a while you just say to yourself, "Oh God, I'm so tired of working out!" You end up hating the gym. Though not necessarily hating activity. I like to move my body, but it took me awhile to find something I would stick to on a regular basis. I had to find a routine that would work for my lifestyle.

Probably the best change I made was to put a treadmill in my bedroom. My wife hates it, and I don't really love having this bulky machine in my room, but when I get out of bed every morning, I have to walk by it. It's right there staring at me, going, "Come here. You know you need this." That makes the ugliness worth it. I usually get on the treadmill for thirty-five to forty-five minutes a day, though on other days I walk outside. But, either way, I do it! The consistency is what it's all about. It's not about becoming some yoga master, gymnast, or bodybuilder. It's about doing something to get your blood flowing, your heart pumping, and your calories burning.

For a long time, exercising was a pretty miserable experience for me. What most people don't understand is that it's very difficult to exercise when you're extremely heavy. You try running around with 350 pounds on you! At that weight I had some back and knee problems, so exercise just didn't feel good. I was caught between a rock and a hard place. I needed to move more to lose the weight, but I couldn't move much because I was so heavy. Exercise felt like punishment.

Except for tennis. I love playing tennis so much that I continued to play it even at my heaviest. I did try to do some other types of exercise too, especially after I first got diagnosed with diabetes, but I have a rebellious streak in me. Being told that I had to go to the gym worked for a while, but it also made activity seem like punishment. And I guess it kind of was. I had slacked off for too long, and now I had to play catch up.

I don't think I'm alone in having regarded exercise as punishment. Tennis has always worked for me because I don't look at it as exercise. I started playing tennis with friends when I was in college. I didn't play in tournaments or anything, but it was competitive. Like poker. You play for bragging rights, dude! It's fun. It's not a chore. I've also learned to love—let me rephrase that—to like the treadmill. Going to the gym, though, wasn't fun for me. It's easy to feel self-conscious with all those slim gym rats around you, and you must always conform to the gym's schedule—another reason it was difficult for me to keep going. Over the years, I had stopped and started going to the gym a hundred times over, but when my health crisis hit, I knew I had to find some way to exercise consistently. I had to take a long hard look at what I could fit into my life and, just as important, what I liked to do.

The pleasure part is critical because it provides an immediate payoff. One reason many people give up on exercise is that they don't see immediate results. You're fifty or one hundred pounds overweight, you start working out, and guess what? It ain't gonna come off right away. This is why people join a gym every January and by March they've stopped showing up. They haven't transformed their bodies, so why bother?

But if you hang in there, great things can happen. A friend of mine started walking ten minutes a day—that's less than a mile, the distance of a lap around most malls. Two weeks later he upped it to eleven minutes, two weeks after that to twelve. He now walks about five miles day, and he lost 125 pounds over the course of a year. If you can get up to walking five miles a day, you're going to be okay.

But it takes patience, and you have to have the tenacity to stay with it until your fitness level improves and the weight comes off. It's work, and, just like my friend, it may take you a whole year. But if you can find a way to make it enjoyable, it's a lot easier to hang in there. Plus, be aware that things are happening. You might not look in the mirror and see a whole new body, but if you are working out regularly, you're going to be stronger, your heart and lung function will have improved, and you'll be more efficient at pumping blood to your muscles. You will also feel better after you get your body moving. Even if you don't love it while it's happening, you're going to be in a better mood and feel more energetic after it's over (and not because the discomfort stops, but because exercise actually alters your brain chemistry). All in all, when you exercise regularly you will be healthier. That's why we're doing this, isn't it?

Health experts recommend that you do both cardiovascular exercise (the kind that increases your heart and breathing rate) and some resistance training, whether it is with weights or bands or using your own body weight (such as doing push-ups and sit-ups). That's ideal. I now do both: every day some cardio exercise (walking or tennis or both), and once or twice a week strength training with free weights (I have a little setup in my garage). Strength training helps control blood sugar, so it's an especially good choice for people who, like me, have diabetes or are at risk for the disease. Training with free weights is really simple. They're cheap and you can buy them at any sporting goods store.

I definitely encourage you to do cardiovascular exercise and strength training if you can, but I also encourage you not to get hung up on any one prescription. What's most important is that you just get your body moving, and there are a lot of ways to do that.

When you hear the word "exercise," traditional activities probably spring to mind: walking, running, swimming, biking, and the gym machines like the elliptical trainer and stair machine. They all provide excellent ways to get fit, but if they totally turn you off, look beyond them. There really are a million activities out there, from ice skating, in-line skating, rowing, and paddle tennis to water aerobics, kickboxing, and basketball. Maybe you like bowling; maybe you like ballet or volleyball. There are hundreds of exercise DVDs out there; there's got to be one routine that you'll like. There's something for everyone.

Exercise for you might be playing with your kids. Find a way of moving that you like, and do it as often as you can. I don't care what you do; just do something.

Get active. And do it every day. That's why walking works so well for me. Since I can do it anywhere, from the comfort of my bedroom to the streets around my office, walking is my mainstay. Every day I decide when I'm going to walk, just like I decide what I'm going to wear. Walking was also the easiest type of exercise for me when I was really heavy. It didn't pound on my joints the way running would have.

I think in my football days I would have laughed at the idea of walking. Real men don't walk! But I've grown to love it (still hate hiking, though). When I'm doing it on the treadmill, I can watch TV, read the newspaper (tricky but possible), talk on the phone. When I'm doing it outside, I find it's a good time just to think, plain and simple. I get ideas, work out problems in my head, and sometimes even experience a shift in my way of thinking. Move a muscle, change a thought! It is, of course, a great time to listen to music too (you'll find my favorite play-lists on page 191).

You don't have to have someplace special to walk. Walk around your block ten times or up and down your street twenty times. If your hood doesn't feel safe, go somewhere else and walk. Go to a park in a safer neighborhood, get to work early and walk around that area, or walk around the mall. At this point, mall walking has become kind of a cliché, but it is abso-lutely a great choice for anyone looking for a safe place to move her body. If you're motivated, you can find a place to walk that's out of harm's way. And if you're really motivated, you can find people to walk with, whether it's a friend, a group of friends, or a walking club.

A lot of health groups recommend that you exercise three to four days a week. Maybe that's because that's all they think most people will do. The reality of it is that if you're trying to lose weight, that's not enough. You have to get up and move every day. Maybe some days you'll do a formal workout and others you'll just play around. Sometimes my exercise for the day is shooting hoops or throwing the football with my kids. Just try to do something daily. Don't con yourself into thinking that a day off is no big deal. One day so easily becomes three. By the same token, don't beat yourself up because you were too tired to exercise or life got in the way of your workout time. Just realize that you've got to get back to it right away. Be unwavering in your commitment to activity and your body will benefit.

A Four-Phase Workout Plan

As you now know, I advocate walking. If you can get to the point where you are doing that regularly, baby, that's all you need. *But,* if you can work up to doing more, you're the bomb! Definitely go for it. Even if you're not feeling it right now, once you start getting stronger and healthier you might be up for the challenge. And if you are, I have a step-by-step plan to get you there.

To pull this plan together, I talked to three of the best trainers I know: Catherine Chiarelli, Brittania Erickson, and Tarik Tyler, the experts I introduced on page xxxi. Now, while I've gone to trainers for their fitness ideas, I'm not sending you to boot camp. Instead, I asked Catherine, Brittania, and Tarik this:

"What can someone do to get fit that doesn't require going to a gym or involve much expense or fancy equipment?" "What," I asked, "is absolutely simple? What is absolutely easy?"

The answers they gave me form the four-phase workout plan on the upcoming pages. It starts with Phase One, a set of stretches and easy strengtheners designed to get your body moving and your blood flowing. Phase Two is walking. Just walking, plain and simple. Phase Three is a group of resistance-training exercises that you can add to your regimen if you want to gain more strength and muscle tone. Phase Four is a circuit-training plan, a kill-two-birds-with-one-stone workout that combines cardio and strength training.

Do one of these phases, do two, or do all of them. It doesn't matter as long as you do something—and stay with it!

Let me add this: lack of time is the biggest excuse people give for not exercising. Don't tell me you don't have the time. You can make the time for something as important as your health. There is probably a gap in your schedule when you are idling—grab that time and use it wisely. If you take your kids to activities, go out and walk while you wait for them. Don't have a drink with a friend, take a walk with a friend. Use your lunch hour as a time to walk (half hour for eating, half hour for walking). If you can't get out of the house, see if you can buy a treadmill (check Craigslist and other classifieds—people are always getting rid of unused exercise equipment). Then get on it while you're watching *American Idol* and other TV shows!

If it's going to make it happen for you, moving's got to be fun. If I said to you, "Hey, you want to go to a party? There's going to be a DJ and dancing." Most people would say yes.

"Do you want to go to the gym and work out?" Most people would say no. So it's not necessarily that they don't like to move, it just has to seem like something other than work for them. If that's you, find your perfect distraction—music is always my top choice—and find an activity you like. If not walking or doing any of the workouts on these pages, then try salsa or ballroom dancing. Check out community college, parks and recreation, and YMCA classes. They all tend to be less expensive and have less of a competitive vibe than gyms, and you can get some great individual attention from the instructors. See what's out there, choose something, and stick with it.

Phase One

Get Pumped: Moves to Get Your Mojo Working

There are a lot of mornings when my treadmill beckons and I just roll over and groan. "Oh, come on—not today, man!" When I know I've got to start walking but my body is objecting, I'll often do a few stretches and easy strengtheners to get it primed for moving. It's amazing how a little movement can change your mind. "Especially in the morning when you're stiff and sleepy, stretching gets your blood flowing, warms you up, and gives you some energy," says Catherine.

The following moves are not only good for shaking off morning stupor, they're a good way to ease into more regular exercise. If you haven't been doing any activity for a long time, this is a good place to start. Try them for a few weeks, then move on to walking or another type of cardiovascular exercise. Your mission is to move, and these simple exercises can help.

One thing to remember is that you don't ever want to do any deep stretching without warming up for five or ten minutes first. However, these stretches are easy, designed just to boost your circulation, increase your flexibility, and get you in the mood for more activity.

<u>WAKE-UP STRETCH</u>
Allover body warm-up

1. Stand with your feet hip-width apart. In one continuous movement, inhale and raise your arms above your head, then exhale, bend your knees, and drop your butt as if you were going to sit in a chair (only go as low as you can without putting too much pressure on your knees).

2. Inhale and return to standing as you bend your arms at a 90-degree angle and pull them back down, elbows by your sides. Do this six times, exhaling as you bend your knees, and inhaling as you straighten your legs and pull your elbows to your sides. When you bend, never allow your knees to go past your ankles.

<u>SEATED HIP STRETCH</u>
Stretches hips, glutes (butt muscles), and hamstrings (backs of thighs)

1. Sit on a chair with your feet flat on the floor, arms down at your sides. Place the outside of your right ankle on your left knee (your legs will form a 4).

2. Inhale, then exhale and fold your upper body over

your legs until you feel a stretch in your right hip, buttocks, and hamstrings. Keep both buttocks evenly on the chair. Let your head drop gently and you will also feel a nice stretch through your neck and down your spine. For a deeper stretch, bring your arms forward over your legs. Hold for fifteen to thirty seconds, breathing as you stretch. Repeat on the other side.

CAT STRETCH WITH BALANCE

Stretches upper and lower back, warming up the spine; works abdominal muscles

1. Get on all fours, thighs and arms perpendicular to the floor and parallel to each other, your wrists directly under your shoulders, and your back straight. Keep your head in line with your spine so that both are parallel to the floor. This is neutral position.

2. Inhale and slowly arch your back and look up slightly, allowing your neck to gently stretch. Inhale four counts up, then exhale for four counts as you tilt your pelvis and round your back, allowing your head to drop as you go. Repeat four times. Return to neutral position.

3. Exhale, lift your right arm and your left leg so that they are straight and parallel to the floor and you are balancing on your left hand and right knee. Pull your abdominal muscles in toward your spine so your belly is strong. Hold for ten counts, breathing in the position. Switch sides. Repeat four times.

PLANK
Strengthens your core, arms, and abdominal muscles

1. Get down on all fours. Raise your knees so that your body is parallel to the floor and you are in the "up" part of a push-up. Keep your head in line with your spine. Your weight should be distributed evenly between your arms and feet.

2. Inhale and exhale as you pull your abdominal muscles in toward your spine. Hold for ten counts, breathing in the position, then release your knees down to the floor and end in child's pose (see below). Repeat four times.

Modification: If it's difficult to achieve the plank position, get down on all fours, then place your forearms on the floor and move forward slightly so that your body is at a forty-five-degree angle. Your elbows should be under your shoulders and your weight evenly distributed between your forearms and feet. If this is difficult to feel, try staying high up on the balls of your feet and extending your heels behind you. As you gain strength, do the exercise with straight arms.

CHILD'S POSE
Stretches back and shoulders

1. Kneel on the ground with your feet together and your knees about hip-width apart. Sit back on your heels and allow your torso to fold over in between your thighs or as low as you can comfortably go. Place your forehead on the floor. Lay your arms on either side of your torso with your palms up, or extend your arms straight in front of you, stretching your shoulders.

2. Let the weight of your shoulders pull you down into a comfortable stretch. Hold for one minute or longer as you breathe slowly and deeply.

MOUNTAIN CLIMBER
Strengthens the core

1. From plank position, pull your abdominal muscles in toward your spine.

2. Inhale, then exhale and bring your right knee toward your chest. Keep you head and neck in line with your spine. Pause, then return to plank and switch sides. Repeat four times. To increase the difficulty of this move, drop your head, round your back, and bring your right knee in as close to your forehead as possible. As you go, your navel should pull in toward your spine and your weight will move slightly forward.

SPINAL TWIST
Stretches upper back, lower back, and hips

1. Lie face up on the floor. Place your arms out to the side, palms flat on the floor. Cross your right leg over your left thigh, knee bent and right foot placed either next to your left knee or hooked under your left calf.

2. Exhale and drop your right leg to the left, aiming your knee toward the floor. Don't force it—it's not important to get your knee to the floor. Keep both shoulders on the floor and turn your head to the right. Hold for thirty seconds to one minute. Repeat on the other side.

Better Than a Coffee Break

When you begin to slump midday, instead of reaching for a cup of coffee try reaching for the sky. "Putting your body through a few moves will fire you back up again without all that caffeine," says Catherine. Here are a few stretches to try.

- To loosen up your shoulders and chest, stand in a doorway, put your arms out to the side, and grasp the door frame slightly lower than shoulder height. Let your body fall slightly forward, until you feel a good stretch across the front of your shoulders and chest. Hold for thirty seconds. Alternative: Clasp your hands behind your back and raise them up toward your shoulders. Hold for thirty seconds. Either one of these exercises will help heighten your awareness of your shoulders throughout the day and keep you from letting them fall forward. That will improve your posture.

- To stretch the back and neck, stand with your legs slightly more than hip-width apart. Roll your head forward, followed by your shoulders and back. Let your upper body hang over your lower body. You can reach for the floor, bend your elbows, and grasp each one with the opposite hand, or rest your hands on your thighs. Breathe in this position for fifteen to thirty seconds, then bend your knees slightly and roll back up through the spine. Allow your head to come up last.

- To stretch hips, glutes, and hamstrings, do the seated hip stretch (page 160).

- To limber up ankles, from seated-hip-stretch position, slide your right leg slightly to the left so that your ankle is beyond your left knee. Circle your ankle to the left ten times, then to the right ten times. Repeat on the other side.

- To work the glutes: sitting on a chair, squeeze the muscles in your butt, hold for ten seconds, and release. Do ten times.

Phase Two

Walking: The Anytime, Anywhere Workout

The reason I love walking so much is because I know I can do it anywhere. When we travel to all those cities, searching for *American Idol* contestants, the days are really long. We'll be in those little audition rooms for ten to twelve hours, with just a few short breaks before finally heading out for a group dinner. During the breaks I try to move my body a little, but I mainly rely on the hotel gym. Dude, I can't flake out! There's just no acceptable excuse. Remember when you travel that just about every hotel has, if not a fully outfitted fitness center, at least a room with a couple of exercise machines.

The thing about being a walker, too, is that besides being able to do it almost anywhere, you can do it in bits and pieces.

If you can't go out and walk for thirty to forty-five minutes straight, you can get in ten minutes here, ten minutes there. That might mean you park ten minutes from your destination and walk to and fro (that's twenty minutes right there). Maybe you walk your dog around the block twice, then later walk from store to store as you get your errands done. Look at life differently, and see where the opportunities to walk lie.

Ideally, though, you'll make the time for several longer sessions per week. If you can do it every day, even better. Here Tarik has some advice on how to get started and how to challenge yourself by improving your time, distance, intensity, or all three.

BEGINNERS GOAL: Walk Two Miles or About Forty Minutes, Three Times a Week

This is a great way to start, but if two miles is difficult for you, just do whatever you can. You'll be amazed at how quickly you gain strength. Keep the pace as brisk as possible, working toward a speed that gets you to break a sweat but still allows you to carry on a conversation.

<u>STEP IT UP</u>

To increase your fitness level and burn more calories, challenge yourself further. There are a few different ways to do this. You can increase the frequency of your walks (this is a good place to start), increase the duration of your walks, or increase their intensity level. Here is how to accomplish each.

Increase frequency: Begin by adding an extra mile, or twenty minutes, of walking on your "off" days. It doesn't have to be a formal workout. You might just park half a mile, or ten minutes, away from work and walk the rest. After two weeks, try to add another formal two-mile/forty-minute workout. Increase your formal workouts every two weeks until you're walking every day.

Increase duration: If you don't have time to walk every day, you can get in more workout time by simply lengthening the duration of your sessions. (And even if you do walk every day, putting in more time on each occasion is a great goal to set your sights on.) As soon as you are up to a solid twenty minutes, start adding five minutes per week. Time is usually an easier way to measure your progress, but if you prefer, you can also use distance as your unit of measure. In that case, increase a quarter of a mile each week.

Increase intensity: Your initial goal, as noted, should be to get up to a brisk pace. From there, try some faster intervals. Use the first five minutes of your walk to warm up, then alternate two minutes of brisk walking with thirty seconds of either very fast walking or jogging. As you get used to the intervals, play with it. See what you can do. Maybe you can bump it up to two minutes of brisk walking, then one minute of fast walking or jogging. This will not only increase your fitness but keep the workout interesting too.

Staying Motivated: You Can't Get Fit If You Quit

The qualities that separate the top *Idol* contestants from the also-rans are perseverance, tenacity, and conviction. But it's not just *Idol*. Everyone who is successful in life, no matter what area they're accomplished in, has those qualities. That's what propels you forward.

The other quality successful people have is that they don't make excuses for themselves. That's something to consider in regard to exercise, because if there is anything that brings out the rationalizer in us, it's exercise. There's *always* an excuse not to do it. The other day a woman said to me, referring to another woman, "Well, she looks like that because she runs five miles a day. I don't like running." I'm thinking to myself, "Okay, here we go." She seemed to be saying that she couldn't lose weight because she doesn't like running. Well, how about walking? Or swimming? I don't care if it's badminton or beach volleyball. Something! I could see that it was a classic case of excuse making.

And I know from excuse making, because I was a world-class excuse maker. So what I did, once I became committed to getting healthy, was to try and remove as many of those potential excuses as possible. For instance, when I wake up and see my treadmill staring me in the face I've got very little justification for not exercising. It's hot out, it's cold out, it's raining—none of that is going to wash.

So okay, there are going to be days when you'll want to dump your exercise routine or just take the easy (or should I say the easy chair) way out. Well, hold steady. Here are some tips to help.

- Revisit your initial reasons for becoming more active. Maybe you just want to feel better. "Think about when you walk through an airport terminal to get to your gate and how nice it would be to get there without being out of breath and sweaty," says Janeen Locker, PhD, the clinical psychologist who you'll be hearing more from in the following chapter. "When you exercise, you're doing something proactive."

- Don't underestimate what your body can do. "A lot of people shortchange themselves when it comes to fitness because maybe they were the last guy picked for the team or the girl with two left feet," says Tarik. "It doesn't matter. You are capable of getting stronger, increasing your stamina, and bettering your coordination. Know that if you pace yourself, your body will improve, and when it does, you're going to feel great about what you've accomplished."

- Have a plan. Don't leave exercise to chance. Know what you're going to do and when you're going to do it. Put it in your calendar as you would any other appointment.

- Have a contingency plan. What are you going to do if it's prohibitively cold outside or raining? "This is when you take your walk to the mall, pop in an exercise DVD, or just do some jumping jacks and jogging in place at home," says Brittania. Find a set of indoor stairs and go up and down them ten times. Put your bike on one of those contraptions that turns it into a stationary cycle.

Maybe during the winter season you take a fitness class and resume walking outdoors in the spring. Be creative and find solutions instead of just giving in to circumstances.

- Set goals that don't relate to your weight. It might be something small (increasing your walking time from fifteen to fourteen minutes per mile), medium (walking a 10 K), or big (entering a marathon). Whatever. Have a goal and work to achieve it.

- Acknowledge, then hold on to, your accomplishments. Give yourself credit for each little goal you achieve. But don't forget that fitness is ephemeral: it will slip away if you don't stick with it. So if, say, you worked hard to get up to doing ten push-ups, don't let that effort go to waste by quitting. You'll just have to do the hard work all over again to get back to ten. Maintain your gains.

- If you tend to be social, find a partner. Having someone to exercise with will make the effort much more pleasurable, and you will also have someone to whom you'll have to be accountable. No getting away with slacking, either of you.

- If you're not social, choose exercise that doesn't require depending on anybody and where you can get some alone time. Walk where you can be anonymous, of try swimming—it's hard for anyone to bother you while you're submerged.

- Broaden your horizons. If your workout isn't making you

happy, find another one that does. It's important to find something you like, and if, okay, you're never going to like exercise, then at least find something you can tolerate. (Again, walking. Who can't tolerate walking?)

• Get back up on the horse. Exercise is like eating. If you have a bad day, don't let it turn into a running disaster. Instead of letting a skipped workout turn into a week of no activity, restart your routine immediately.

Phase Three

Basic Strength Training

There are a lot of reasons to perform a simple strength-training routine a few times a week. Building muscle helps reduce the risk of osteoporosis, counters aging, and boosts your metabolic rate so you burn more calories. Strength training also has a positive impact on blood sugar, good news for diabetics like me as well as for people who are prediabetic. Research shows that combining strength training with cardiovascular exercise is even better: together the two control blood sugar levels more than either one alone.

The strength-training exercises Tarik recommends are very basic. For beginners he offers a quick three-move routine that requires no dumbbells. The intermediate routine adds weights, but takes only about twenty minutes. The exercises work all the big muscles of the body and strengthen your core (the abdominal and back muscles), which can help improve your posture. The only equipment you need is dumbbells. Choose weights that are light enough to allow you do to twelve to fifteen repetitions but heavy enough so that you can barely lift those last few reps. Make sure all your movements are slow and controlled.

Even if you can only do this workout one day a week, it's going to help you get fitter. But aim big. "Three times a week is optimal," says Tarik.

Beginner's Routine

Here are three exercises you can do that don't require any equipment, only your own body weight. As you get stronger, move on to the weight workout.

<u>SQUATS</u>

Strengthens the muscles in the front of the thighs (quads), back of thighs (hamstrings), and buttocks (glutes)

1. Stand with your feet slightly wider than shoulder-width apart, your back straight, head up, and your toes and knees pointed slightly out. There should be a slight bend in your knees.

2. Pull your abdominal muscles in toward your spine. Exhale, bend your knees, and with your upper body leaning slightly forward, lower yourself down until your thighs are almost parallel to the floor. If going that low is difficult, just go as low as you can. Inhale and return to the starting position. Do twelve to fifteen repetitions.

LEANING PLANK UP AND DOWNS
Strengthens the arms and chest

1. Stand straight with your feet hip-width apart, facing a wall about two feet in front of you. Lean in until you are at a steep angle against the wall, bend your elbows and place your forearms on the wall.

2. Exhale and push back; straighten your arms and place your palms flat on the wall. Bend your elbows again and return to starting position. Do twelve to fifteen repetitions.

TRICEP DIPS
Strengthens the backs of the arms (triceps)

1. Stand with your back close to a bench or chair. Bend your knees, lower your body, and, with your arms behind you, grasp the edge of the bench with your palms. Move your legs out as necessary so that your knees are bent at a ninety-degree angle, feet flat on the floor.

2. Exhale and lower your body until your arms are bent at a ninety-degree angle. Inhale and push back up until your arms are straight but not locked. Do twelve to fifteen repetitions.

Modification: If this is too difficult, use a counter or shelf in a bookcase that comes to about midback height instead of a bench, and do the exercise while standing.

Intermediate

DUMBBELL SQUATS

Follow the instructions on page 172, adding dumbbells: hold a dumbbell in each hand, arms at your sides and palms facing inward toward your legs.

LUNGES

Strengthens the muscles in the thighs (hamstrings and quadriceps) and buttocks (glutes)

1. Stand with your right foot in front of your left foot, about a few inches farther than one stride's length apart. Hold a dumbbell in each hand, arms at your sides and palms facing inward toward your legs.

2. Pull your abdominal muscles in toward your spine, exhale, and bend both knees, allowing your left heel to come up in back and your front thigh to become as close to parallel to the floor as possible. Your front knee should be directly above your ankle—never beyond it. Pause, inhale, and rise up. Do twelve to fifteen repetitions. Switch sides.

SHOULDER PRESSES

Strengthens shoulders and backs of upper arms (triceps)

1. Sit in a chair with your feet flat on the floor. Pull in your abdominal muscles to keep your back flat against the back of the chair.

2. Holding a dumbbell in each hand, raise your arms in

front of you to shoulder level, elbows bent, palms facing forward. Exhale and raise the dumbbells overhead until your arms are almost straight (don't lock your elbows) and the inside ends of the dumbbells are nearly touching each other. Pause for a second, then inhale and slowly lower the dumbbells to the starting position. Do twelve to fifteen repetitions.

<u>ONE-ARM ROW</u>
Strengthens back and shoulders

1. Kneel on a bench with your left leg and place your left arm in front of your knee, palm on the bench. Your right foot will be on the floor and your right leg next to the bench, supporting your weight. Hold a dumbbell in your right hand with your arm hanging down, palm facing inward.

2. Pull your abdominal muscles in toward your spine. Exhale, bend your right elbow, and gradually raise the dumbbell up to about chest height. Keep your elbow high and finish above your shoulder. Pause, inhale, and return to the starting position. Do twelve to fifteen repetitions. Switch sides.

<u>FORWARD BICEP CURLS</u>
Strengthens fronts of upper arms (biceps)

1. Stand with your feet hip-width apart, knees slightly bent. Holding a dumbbell in each hand, place your arms close to your body, palms facing out.

2. Exhale, contract your biceps, and raise both dumbbells up to your chest, keeping your upper arms close to your body. Inhale and slowly lower. Do twelve to fifteen repetitions.

TRICEP EXTENSIONS
Strengthens backs of upper arms (triceps)

1. Sit in a chair with your feet flat on the floor. Pull in your abdominal muscles to keep your back flat against the back of the chair. Grasp the rounded end of a dumbbell with both hands and hold it up over and slightly behind your head, arms straight but not locked. The other end of the dumbbell should be pointing down toward the floor.

2. Exhale, bend your elbows, and slowly lower the dumbbell behind your head, keeping your upper arms still. Pause, inhale, and slowly raise the dumbbell back to starting position. Do twelve to fifteen repetitions.

CRUNCHES
Strengthens abdominal muscles

1. Lie on your back, knees bent, feet flat on the floor. Clasp your hands behind your head. Pull your abdominal muscles in toward your spine and flatten your lower back against the floor.

2. Exhale, contract your abdominals, and slowly curl your shoulders and upper back forward. Your neck should be straight and your chin raised. Hold for a few seconds, then inhale and slowly lower down. Do fifteen to twenty repetitions.

LATERAL CRUNCHES
To strengthen the side abdominal muscles (obliques)

1. Lie on your back, knees bent, feet flat on the floor. Clasp your hands behind your head. Let your knees fall to the right, and adjust your hips to get them closer to the floor.

2. Exhale, pull your abdominal muscles in toward your spine, and, keeping your shoulders parallel to the floor, curl your upper body toward your hips. Your neck should be straight and your chin raised. Hold for a second, then inhale and lower down. Do twelve to fifteen repetitions. Switch sides.

PUSH-UPS: BEGINNER
To strengthen the chest and arms

1. Place your hands and knees on the floor, your hands slightly wider than shoulder width. Cross your ankles behind you.

2. Keeping your back straight, inhale, then exhale and bend your elbows to lower your upper body one to two inches from the floor. Inhale and press up with your hands. Do as many repetitions as possible, working up to twelve to fifteen.

PUSH-UPS: ADVANCED

1. Place your hands and knees on the floor with your hands shoulder-width apart. Raise up on your toes and arms. Keep your arms straight but not locked.

2. With your body straight, exhale and bend your elbows to lower your body one or two inches from the floor. Inhale and press up with your hands. Do as many repetitions as possible, working up to twelve to fifteen.

Real-Life Alert
Exercise Makes Me Too Hungry

When you're trying to improve your eating and exercise habits, it's frustrating to find that working out can make it harder to stick to the healthy-eating half of the plan. What I'm talking about are those days when you spend a half hour exercising then come home feeling like you could eat everything in your refrigerator—and sometimes you do. What's going on?

"Exercise will have a subtle effect on your appetite, and there's nothing wrong with feeling hungrier," says Erin. "Just don't overcompensate." There are two reasons why people often feel excessively hungry after exercise. One is that they are working out too hard and not eating enough to keep up with their bodies' need for fuel. The other is more psychological. "You start thinking, I've been good, I've worked out, I can eat," says Erin. Yeah, that sounds familiar. I've been guilty of that.

Here's what can help. Don't put off eating for too long because you know you're going to exercise. It's okay to eat up until twenty to thirty minutes before you work out as long as you eat something easy to digest like a protein bar, banana, or pear (stay away from acidic fruits like apples and oranges, which can cause stomachaches, and high-fiber choices, which take a long time to digest). A piece of toast with a little peanut butter, a small serving of yogurt, or an ounce of cheese are all good choices. If you are going to be working out for longer than an hour, take a snack and water or sports drink along.

After a rigorous workout, eating within the hour can help you repair muscle tissue and replace the glycogen in your muscles (glycogen is stored glucose, the muscles' prime fuel). Choose something that has a mix of carbohydrates, protein, and fat, like all the foods mentioned above. If you have something small to eat within that twenty- to-thirty-minute window, it may also help you ward off an I'm-so-hungry-I-could-eat-a-horse eruption later. Plus: "It's a good time to eat because exercise increases your metabolism. That means you'll utilize the calories you take in more efficiently," says Erin.

While eating smartly before and after exercise may help you avoid diving into the fridge, also realize that being active doesn't give you a pass when it comes to eating right. Stick to the strategies I talk about in chapters 5 and 6 and you'll be less likely to have big hunger swings even after exercise.

Phase Four

Circuit Training: Kicking It Up a Notch

The beauty of a circuit-training workout is that it combines both strength and cardio training. You wipe out your fitness commitment in one fell swoop. The cool thing, too, is that you don't have to go to a gym to do a circuit-training workout. And you need very little equipment: just some dumbbells, though you can also skip the dumbbells if you want and do the strength-training exercises using your own body weight.

Circuit training involves alternating exercises that get your heart rate up with resistance exercises. It's a continuous workout—the exercises flow from one to the other without pause. Brittania designed this particular plan as a mix-and-match workout: she gives you eleven cardio and eighteen strength-training choices. For the best allover workout, you'll want to choose strength-training exercises that hit different areas of the body, but even within those different areas you'll almost always have a choice (there are, for instance, three different exercises for triceps, the muscles in the backs of the arms). You can do this workout differently every time, which means it's a lot less likely that you'll get bored. Here are the specifics.

Thirty-Minute Circuit Workout

This combination workout should take you about thirty minutes, though possibly less, depending on how fit you already are. Thirty minutes! That's nothing. You can do this, dawg. Here's how it works: Survey the lists of cardiovascular exercises and strength-training exercises. Pick two cardio and five strength training (preferably ones that hit a range of body parts). Start with one cardio exercise, then do your first strengthening exercise. Next comes your second cardio choice, then your second strengthening choice. In the third round, go back to your first cardio exercise, but move on to your third strength-training choice. Continue alternating between your two cardio choices until you've done all five strength-training exercises, ending with a cardio pick. (See the sample workout, below.)

Your goal should be to keep moving without taking a break between the cardio and strength-training exercises. It may take you some time to get the routine down, but you'll start remembering the exercises with practice. You may want to start with one circuit, but your goal should be to work up to three.

<u>SAMPLE WORKOUT</u>

Start with a ten- to fifteen-minute walk or with some easy jogging in place to get your body warmed up.

Cardio: jump rope
Strength: shoulder press
Cardio: side shuffle
Strength: forward bicep curl
Cardio: jump rope
Strength: walking lunges
Cardio: side shuffle
Strength: crunches
Cardio: jump rope
Strength: leg lifts
Cardio: side shuffle

Repeat two times for a total of three circuits.

When you finish, finish with a round of stretches. Try doing the wake-up stretch, seated hip stretch, cat stretch (without the balance), child's pose, and spinal twist or a routine of your own. Weight training shortens the muscles, so following with stretches can help you return to your normal and even improve your range of motion.

Cardio Choices

All these moves require momentum. Keep up a good pace. Pick any two.

STEP-UPS

Using a curb or other low step, step up with your left foot then right foot, and then down with left, down with right. Repeat, leading with the other foot. Do twenty times, alternating feet.

SIDE SHUFFLE

Take a wide step to the side with one foot, then bring the other foot to meet it. As soon as your feet touch, move to the next step. Shuffle a distance of about ten feet, ten to twenty times.

JUMP ROPE

Jump with an actual rope or go through the motion without a rope, twenty to fifty times.

JUMPING JACKS

Stand with your hands at your sides, then simultaneously jump your feet apart and clap your hands together above your head. Do twenty to fifty times.

HIGH KNEES

Run in place, exaggerating the height of your knees by pulling them up toward your chest. Do twenty times.

BUTT KICKS

Run in place, exaggerating the height of your feet by trying to kick your butt as you go. Do twenty times.

BURPEES

Squat down and put your hands flat on the floor in front of you. Walk or jump your feet back so that you are in a push-up position, then walk or jump your feet back to your hands and stand up. Do five to ten times.

SCISSOR JUMPING JACKS

Stand with feet together. Jump your right foot back and your left foot forward. Raise your right arm forward and left arm back at shoulder height as you go (the arms follow the feet). Do twenty to fifty times.

KNEE LIFTS

Using a curb or other low step, step up with your left foot, raise your right knee toward your chest, then step down. Repeat on the other side. Do twenty times, alternating feet.

JUMP SQUATS

From a standing position, squat then jump up. Do five to fifteen times.

JUMP SQUATS WITH PUNCHES

From a standing position, squat, jump up, then land back in standing position and do four boxing punches with knees slightly bent (as you get stronger, you can add light dumbbells). Do ten times.

Modification: If jumping is too high impact, raise up on your toes as you do the boxing punches instead.

Strength-Training Choices

Some of the following exercises can be done with dumbbells or not. Your choice. If you are using weights, choose lighter ones that will allow you to do fifteen to twenty repetitions. By the end of those fifteen or twenty reps, you should barely be able to lift the weight. As a general rule, exhale on the exertion and inhale as you release. Also work these exercises in a slow and controlled fashion so you get maximum benefit.

Pick five.

Abdominals
CRUNCHES
See page 176. Do fifteen to twenty repetitions.

LEG RAISES

1. Lie on your back and slide your hands under your butt, palms down. Raise your legs to a ninety-degree angle.

2. Pull your abdominal muscles in toward your spine so

that your back is flat against the floor. Exhale and lower your legs two to three inches from the floor. Don't allow your back to arch as your legs lower. Inhale and raise your legs back up. Do fifteen to twenty repetitions. If you can only lower your legs a quarter of the way, start with that. As you gain strength you'll be able to lower them farther.

SEATED TWIST

1. Sit on the floor with your knees bent, feet flat, back straight. Clasp your hands in front of your chest, elbows out to the side.

2. Pull your abdominal muscles in toward your spine, exhale, and slowly twist to the right. Inhale and return to center. Repeat on the other side. Do fifteen to twenty repetitions. As you get stronger, do the exercise leaning back with your torso at a forty-five-degree angle.

Core (Abdominal Muscles and Lower Back)
PLANK
See page 162. Do fifteen to twenty repetitions.

BRIDGES

1. Lie on the floor with your knees bent, feet flat on the floor. Place your hands by your sides, palms down.

2. Exhale and raise your pelvis, pressing down on your arms and feet to help you. When you are up as far as you can go, squeeze your butt and slowly lower down. Don't bounce. Do fifteen to twenty repetitions.

SUPERMANS

1. Lie on your stomach, nose to the ground, with your arms stretched out above your head.

2. Exhale and raise your upper and lower body simultaneously. Hold for a second, then lower down. Do fifteen to twenty repetitions.

Modification: If it's too tough to raise both your upper and lower body, do a set where you raise your upper body, then do a set raising your lower body. Work up to raising both together.

Back and Shoulders
BOXING PUNCHES

1. Stand with your right leg forward and your left leg about a foot behind it. Bend your knees slightly. Raise your hands in a boxer's stance.

2. Alternate punching left and right, using your legs to give you power. Do two sets of twenty punches.

Shoulders
SHOULDER PRESSES
See page 174. Do fifteen to twenty repetitions.

ARM CIRCLES

1. Stand with your feet about hip-width apart. Holding a dumbbell in each hand, reach your arms out to the sides at shoulder level. (The dumbbells are optional.)

2. Circle your arms forward twenty times. Reverse and circle your arms backward twenty times.

Chest
PUSH-UPS
See page 177. Do fifteen to twenty repetitions.

CHEST PRESSES

1. Lie on your back with your knees bent, feet flat on the floor. Pull in your abdominal muscles so that your back lies flat. Hold a dumbbell in each hand, arms out to the side at shoulder level and bent at a ninety-degree angle.

2. Keeping your abdominal muscles firm, exhale and slowly raise both dumbbells up until your arms are straight but not locked. Pause for a second, then slowly return the dumbbells back to the starting position. Do fifteen to twenty repetitions.

Biceps (Fronts of Upper Arms)
FORWARD BICEP CURLS
See page 175. Do fifteen to twenty repetitions.

HAMMER BICEP CURLS

1. Stand with your knees slightly bent, feet hip-width apart. Holding a dumbbell in each hand, place your arms close to your body, palms toward your legs.

2. Exhale, contract your biceps, and raise both dumbbells up to your chest, keeping your upper arms close to your body. Inhale and slowly lower. Do fifteen to twenty repetitions.

REVERSE BICEP CURLS

1. Stand with your knees slightly bent, feet hip-width apart. Holding a dumbbell in each hand, place your arms close to your body, palms facing behind you.

2. Exhale, contract your biceps, and as you raise both dumbbells up to your chest twist your arms so that you end up with your palms facing toward your shoulders (keep your upper arms close to your body as you go). Inhale and slowly lower. Do fifteen to twenty repetitions.

Triceps (backs of upper arms)
LYING TRICEP EXTENSION

1. Lie on your back. Grasp the rounded end of a dumbbell with both hands and hold the dumbbell above your forehead, with arms straight but not locked.

2. Exhale and slowly lower the dumbbell behind your head, allowing it to touch the ground. Pause for a second, inhale, and slowly press it back up over your forehead.

TRICEP EXTENSIONS
See page 176. Do fifteen to twenty repetitions.

TRICEP DIPS
See page 173. Do fifteen to twenty repetitions.

Calves
CALF RAISES

1. Stand with your feet hip-width apart, a dumbbell in each hand, palms facing inward toward your legs. (The dumbbells are optional.)

2. Exhale and raise up on the toes of your right foot. Do fifteen to twenty repetitions. Switch sides. Repeat, raising up on both toes at the same time.

Modification: If balance is an issue for you, forgo the dumbbells and hold on to a stair rail.

Thighs
WALKING LUNGES

1. Stand with your feet hip-width apart, a dumbbell in each hand, palms facing inward toward your legs. (The dumbbells are optional.)

2. Exhale and step forward with your right foot, bending both knees so that your right knee is at a ninety-degree angle and your left knee points toward the floor (your front foot will be flat on the ground; you'll be on your toes in back, upper body straight).

3. Inhale, straighten your legs, and step forward with your left foot, repeating the lunge on the other side. Do ten to fifteen repetitions on each side.

LUNGES WITH KNEE RAISE

1. Stand with your feet hip-width apart, a dumbbell in each hand, palms facing inward toward your legs. (The dumbbells are optional.)

2. Exhale and in one smooth motion raise your right knee to your chest, then bring it behind you as you bend your left knee into a lunge position (your front foot will be flat on the ground; you'll be on your toes in back, upper body straight).

3. Return to starting position and repeat on the other side. Do fifteen to twenty repetitions on each side.

Work Out, Rock Out

Sometimes I get so lost in the music I'm listening to that I don't even notice that I've been working out for a half hour. Occasionally I even get so into it that I go way beyond the time I set out to exercise for. Music makes pumping the treadmill (or whatever you do) a lot easier and a lot more enjoyable. And that's not just in my own experience. Studies have shown that people work out longer and harder when they listen to music. Music, to be sure, is a great distraction and a great motivator.

I love all kinds of tunes from hip-hop to country so I really mix up the play list on my iPod. Here are three collections of songs (all available on iTunes) that I recommend trying out; they're as energizing as they are eclectic.

PLAY LIST 1

"Dance Like There's No Tomorrow"—Paula Abdul

"Dance Like There's No Tomorrow"—Paula Abdul (Paul Oakenfold Remix)

"Lets Go to Bed"—The Cure

"Being a Girl"—Van Hunt

"Start Me Up"—The Rolling Stones

"Good Life"—Kanye West

"Breathe Me"—Sia

"Fly Away"—Lenny Kravitz

"Don't Stop 'Til You Get Enough" —The Jacksons

"California Love"—Zapp & Roger

"Golden Slumbers/Carry the Weight"—Paul McCartney

"Clocks"—Coldplay

"All the Small Things"—Blink-182

"Make It Happen"—Mariah Carey

"Jump"—Kris Kross

"SexyBack"—Justin Timberlake

"At the End of a Slow Dance"—Van Hunt

"My Humps"—Black Eyed Peas

"Buttons"—The Pussycat Dolls

"Don't Cha"—The Pussycat Dolls

"Hey Ya!"—OutKast

"Addicted to Love"—Robert Palmer

"Beat It"—Fall Out Boy featuring John Mayer

"Crazy"—Gnarls Barkley

"Born for This"—Paramore

"Call Me"—Blondie

"Chains of Love"—Erasure

"Chasing Cars"—Snow Patrol

"See You Again"—Miley Cyrus

"Damaged"—Danity Kane

"Dance to the Music"—Sly & the Family Stone

"Boulevard of Broken Dreams"—Green Day

PLAY LIST 2

"I Would Die 4 You"—Prince

"Don't Stop Believin' "—Journey

"Everybody Got Their Something"—Nikka Costa

"Fade Into You"—Mazzy Star

"Family Affair"— Joss Stone and Sly & the Family Stone

"High Time for Getting Down"—Travis Tritt

"The South's Gonna Do It Again"—Charlie Daniels

"I Got a Woman"—Ray Charles

"Nine in the Afternoon"—Panic at the Disco

"I Write Sins Not Tragedies"—Panic! at the Disco

"Low"—Flo Rida featuring T-Pain

"In Love with a Girl"—Gavin DeGraw

"It Ends Tonight"—The All-American Rejects

"It's Goin' Down"—Yung Joc

"It's the Same Old Song"—Boyz II Men

"Jolene"—Dolly Parton

"Jump Around"—House of Pain

"Kiss Kiss"—Chris Brown featuring T-Pain

"Beautiful Girls"—Sean Kingston

"Love Don't Live Here"—Lady Antebellum

"Madly"—Tristan Prettyman

"Makes Me Wonder"—Maroon 5

"Misery Business"—Paramore

"Money (That's What I Want)"—Boyz II Men

"Rehab"—Amy Winehouse, remix featuring Jay-Z

"The Scientist"—Coldplay

"Feels Just Like It Should"—Jamiroquai

"Shawty Get Loose"—Lil Mama

"Simply Irresistible"—Robert Palmer

"Don't Stop the Music"—Rihanna

"Speed of Sound"—Coldplay

"Unforgettable"—Nat King Cole

"Hallelujah"—Jeff Buckley

PLAY LIST 3

"Unfinished Symphony"—Massive Attack

"We Takin' Ova"—DJ Khaled featuring Rick Ross, Fat Joe, Akon, TI, Baby, Lil Wayne

"Hey! Bo Diddley"—Bo Diddley

"You're Still the One"—Shania Twain

"4 Minutes"—Madonna, featuring Justin Timberlake and Timbaland

"Bleeding Love"—Leona Lewis

"Lollipop"—Lil Wayne

"Shake It"—Metro Station

"Before He Cheats"—Carrie Underwood

"Realize"—Colbie Caillat

"Feels Like Tonight"—Daughtry

"Mercy"—Duffy

"Indestructible"—Disturbed

"Bust It Baby, Pt. 2"—Plies

"Sexy Can I"—Ray J

"She's a Hottie"—Toby Keith

"No Air"—Jordin Sparks and Chris Brown

"Whatever It Takes"—Lifehouse

"When I Grow Up"—The Pussycat Dolls

"Ahora Es"—Wisin & Yandel

"Te Quiero"—Flex, featuring Belinda

"Wonderwall"—Oasis

"Love in This Club"—Usher

"Real Love"—Mary J. Blige

"Dance, Dance, Dance"—Chic

"Hey Baby"—No Doubt, featuring Bounty Killer

Oatmeal Apple Spice Cookies

As cookies go, these are considerably healthier than your average Toll House. The oatmeal, apple, and walnuts all contribute fiber, and applesauce and yogurt add moisture without fat.

Makes about 36 cookies

Have on hand:
cookie sheets
canola oil cooking spray
food processor
sifter
medium mixing bowl
large mixing bowl
electric mixer
wire cooling rack

3 cups old-fashioned rolled oats, divided
1 cup unbleached flour
1 teaspoon baking soda
1/2 teaspoon salt
1 teaspoon ground cinnamon
1 teaspoon ground cloves
1/4 teaspoon ground nutmeg
1 tablespoon light butter
3/4 cup packed brown sugar
1/4 cup sugar
1 egg

½ cup unsweetened applesauce
⅓ cup nonfat plain yogurt
1 Granny Smith apple, peeled and diced
½ cup chopped walnuts*

Preheat oven to 350°F. Lightly spray cookie sheets with canola oil spray, and set aside.

Measure 1 cup of oats and process in a blender to a fine powder. Sift processed oats, unbleached flour, baking soda, salt, and spices into a medium bowl and set aside.

In a large mixing bowl, cream together the butter and sugars until light and fluffy. Beat in the egg, applesauce, and yogurt. Stir in flour mixture, apple, and walnuts until combined.

Drop cookie dough by 1½ tablespoons onto prepared cookie sheets, spaced two inches apart. Bake for 9 to 12 minutes or until cookies start to turn golden on the edges. Cool cookies for 5 minutes, then transfer to wire cooling rack.

Per serving (2 cookies per serving): 162 calories, 4g fat (22.1% calories from fat), 4g protein, 28g carbohydrate, 2g dietary fiber, 14mg cholesterol, 152mg sodium.

*Note: Omitting chopped walnuts from recipe will save 2 grams fat and 21 calories per serving.

CHAPTER EIGHT

Why You Do Those Things You Do

During *Idol* season, Simon, Paula, and I don't have much interaction with the contestants. On purpose. After all, we have to judge them so we shouldn't be telling them what to do beforehand or offering advice beyond what we give in our critiques. But if I were able to talk to them during the competition, I would say this: Get your head in the right place. Don't let the pressure get to you. Just work hard and stay true to yourself.

The pressure is rough on these kids, and for some it's insurmountable. You can see it happening in their defeated faces as they're going out the door. Just having to tough out the judging is difficult enough, but to be going through it on a TV show of *Idol*'s magnitude, with millions of eyeballs on you? That's especially rough. And then, just when you think it can't get any rougher, there are all kinds of blogs, Web sites, and tabloids weighing in, not only on your singing, but on your clothes, your hair, your personality. *What?! They don't even know me.* We often tell stars in the music business not to read their own press. It can wreck you.

The pressure, though, is also part of the competition. Can you stand the heat? If not, get out of the kitchen, baby. Because if you can't deal with the pressure, this business might not be right for you. Madonna doesn't care about the pressure. She thrives on it. Elvis didn't care about the pressure. "They're talking about me?" "Yeah, they're saying that they hate you." "Oh, that's because they actually love me." That's the attitude! Thrive on the pressure.

This is a kind of roundabout way of getting to my next point (yes, I do have one): Common wisdom would have you believe that losing weight is all about how much you eat and how much you move your body. But my experience tells me something different. I think the biggest factor is what's going on in your head. You've got to be psyched up, meaning you've got to be pumped, ready to do it! And you can't let yourself get psyched out, meaning tangled up in the expectations of others or fearful that you don't have what it takes to do it. Trust me, you do.

While I hope that the eating and exercise strategies I laid out in the previous chapters will help you, I also urge you to spend some time thinking honestly about what you really want from life. Before I had my gastric bypass surgery, I had many sessions with a psychologist where we talked about what lay ahead of me after the procedure. It's not like I didn't know that eating with abandon wasn't good for me. But what was going to make me honor that knowledge once I'd risked my life and spent a lot of money to have the surgery? It was essential that I come out of the operation with the right attitude. Unless I changed my way of thinking, all the eating and exercise strategies in the world wouldn't have helped me.

Keeping the Whole Family Healthy

Of all the cool things that have happened to me (and how cool is it to have worked with Bob Dylan and Bruce Springsteen?), one of the coolest was being named Dad of the Month by iParenting.com, a Web site for moms and dads. It was a great compliment, because I'm fiercely devoted to setting my kids on the right path and helping them avoid the family curse of diabetes. Of course, this curse isn't exclusive to my family. Children are being diagnosed with type 2 diabetes in record numbers. It's up to all parents to do what they can to help their kids maintain a healthy body weight, eat right, and exercise. Or I should say, maintain a healthy body weight, eat right, and *play*. Kids don't need to exercise per se, they just need to get out there and run around.

The number one thing you can do for the health of your kids is set a good example. Your kids may seem like they're ignoring you, but don't be fooled. They are watching everything you do. If you eat healthfully and lead an active life, there's a greater chance that they will too. It's not just the foods you put in their lunches or on the dinner table at night, and it's not just the sports you enroll them in (though all those things are important too). What counts more than anything is how good a role model you are. Your kids may not always do what you say, but there's a good chance that they will do what you do.

Getting kids to eat healthfully is a tough job, that's for sure. Kids want to be kids, and I believe we should let them—but within reason. The rule of moderation that I live by is the one I expect my kids to live by too. We don't keep lots of junk in the house; that's way too tempting. At a birthday party, sure, they can have cake and ice cream. I don't want to take one of the fun things in life away from them. I'm not going to keep them from trick-or-treating on Halloween or snatch away the candy when they come home. I know one family whose kids have *never* had sugar. That's cool. But that's not how I'm raising my family. I don't think that approach would work so well in our household. No, we're all about everything in moderation.

And if I did try to forbid sugar, I'm sure they'd go out of their way to get cake, ice cream, and candy somehow. But I don't want my kids to have to sneak around to get all those less-than-stellar foods. I do, however, want them to know that those things are "once in a while" foods. They don't get to eat them every day, and when they do eat them, it should be in reasonably sized portions. For that reason, we stock up on a lot of 100-calorie packs of cookies and chips in our house. The kids don't feel deprived, and we have the comfort of knowing that they're eating the junkier types of food in moderation.

We also rarely go to fast-food restaurants. I know, I know, kids *love* fast food, but it's a terrible habit to cultivate. The National Heart, Lung, and Blood Institute did a study that found that young adults, eighteen to thirty, who ate at fast-food restaurants more than twice a week were in real trouble. As compared to young people who ate fast food only once a week, they were heavier and had a twofold increase in insulin resistance, a risk factor for type 2 diabetes. I don't want to set my kids up for that kind of trouble so early in life.

One of my goals is to help my kids have a healthier relationship with food, and that includes following the advice of diabetes experts like Dr. Fran. She tells parents not to use food to comfort their kids—even though it's something all cultures have done for generations. "When you nurture someone with food, all of a sudden food becomes love," she says, explaining that one reason kids grow up to be adults who overeat is because they use food to soothe themselves. "We need to work on disconnecting the two."

The other side of the coin, of course, is activity. Just like you and me, kids have got to move. As difficult as it is to get kids to eat foods that are good for them, it may be even harder to pull them away from TV, computers, and video games so they'll go outside and play. I used to play all day! Granted, it's not as easy for kids now. Not only do parents feel it's not safe for kids to be roaming around on their bikes like we used to, but the demands of school have increased tremendously. Most kids have little free time. My deal is that you've got to make free time for them. If you are scheduling your kids like there's no tomorrow, at least allow them to spend some of that scheduled time doing something active, be it soccer or swimming or ballet. And when they do have free time, encourage them to run around. If it's not safe in your hood, find a park. I don't care if it's twenty miles across town. Pack a lunch and go as a family, so you can all get some exercise. It comes back to being a good role model. My kids see me walking and playing tennis all the time, and they see Erika, a former dancer, doing her kickboxing. It helps. Get out there and show them how to do it!

Ultimately, weight loss is all about telling yourself the truth. It's about being honest about what you can realistically achieve and what you can live with in terms of eating right and exercising. And it's about being honest about whose struggle this is: it's yours and yours alone. You have to live in your own body and be your own person.

In the introduction, I said that while I was concerned about my family—of course I want to be around to see my children grow up—I knew that this couldn't be about my feelings for anyone else. I had to want to regain my health because of how I felt about *me*. I had to love and respect myself enough to do right by myself. What's more, it was up to me and no one else to take control of my reality.

One question I put to Dr. Locker (see page 204 for more of our discussion and page xxx to learn more about her), was this: "What generally gets people to finally take control of their health?" She agreed that a lot of it has to do with their internal dialogue. "When people finally decide to do something about their health, it's not because an aunt said, 'You need to lose weight,'" says Dr. Locker. "It's usually because they're tired of the mental struggle and they've decided it's time to make a change. They're clear about the fact that they're in control. No one else is going to come in and sweep away the problem. They realize that they have to be willing to make all those mini-decisions throughout the day that contribute to a healthy lifestyle. It's having the focus and drive to say yes or no multiple times a day."

Being real with yourself can be challenging, but learning to handle the truth about your own body and behavior is critical. Not the truth as told to you by judges like me, Simon, and Paula—or your friends or family or even your doctors— the truth told *to* you *by* you. It's you being honest with yourself.

Often the truth isn't pretty. One thing I had to come to terms with was that I was essentially an addict. Like a drug addict, I often needed a momentary high from food. I needed an escape. I used food as a way to enhance or diminish every emotion I experienced. If I was depressed, I hoped that it would provide temporary reprieve. If I was happy, what better way to celebrate? Different people use food in different ways. My problem wasn't that I used food to cope—sitting on the couch with a tub of ice cream because I was sad wasn't my thing.

What I did instead was constantly reward myself with food, no matter what emotional state I was in. This was at the heart of my addiction. Whether it's drugs, alcohol, or food, an addiction is an addiction. And it's okay to admit that you need help with an addiction. Instead of reaching for the chocolate cake, I should have been reaching out to a therapist, asking to sit down and talk.

I am all for finding people who can help you get on track. But I'm also for ultimately becoming your own coach. Take the messages you get from trainers, dietitians, therapists, and other experts and internalize them. You can't have someone holding your hand forever. Resolve to be accountable to yourself.

Happiness, Sadness, Food, and Staying Motivated: A Psychologist Weighs In

As much as I consider myself a student of human nature, I love to hear from people who really are (that is, professionally) students of human nature. One of them is Dr. Locker, who is well versed in the challenges that go with weight loss. We had a conversation about some of the emotional and behavioral issues that crop up when you're trying to improve your health.

RJ: Why do we always love the things that are bad for us? Why do we want to eat everything that's unhealthy? It tastes good, of course, but aren't there reasons beyond that?

Dr. Locker: There can be multiple reasons. One may be that abusing foods allows us to escape ourselves. The self that we put forth to others takes a lot of work and sometimes doesn't reflect the complexity of who we really are. For instance, the daughter who goes to church regularly and does everything else she is supposed to do may feel stifled by that public self and so overeats to fulfill a different aspect of herself. By bingeing she allows that wild side to be expressed. That's one potential reason.

Another is that sometimes people don't think they deserve to feel good. Based on early parent interactions, they may internalize punishment from their parents and reenact this punishment by maybe dieting or forcing themselves to overexercise. But self-punishment doesn't work for long and they end up rebelling against it, potentially by overeating. That sets up a cycle where they are left feeling an emotional hangover of shame and guilt. Eventually it becomes, "This is boring, I want to have that cake. And now I feel awful because I ate too much cake."

RJ: Everyone talks about "emotional eating" and the idea that people who are overweight overeat because they're unhappy or depressed. What do you think?

Dr. Locker: There is a strong connection between food and feelings. Some people overeat because they are excited and happy—despite our cultural stereotype of the depressed, lonely overeater. Some people feel like they are taking in more joy by eating more food.

RJ: Yes! That was me. I'd overeat whether happy or sad.

Dr. Locker: It can work both ways. Some people do eat to help them cope with uncomfortable emotions. If your parents mollified you with food when you were younger, at some point you'll learn to do it yourself. Self-soothing with food can then become your main mechanism for coping with feelings of sadness and loneliness.

The urge to overeat or binge in some cases is a signal that something is not right either internally, within yourself, or externally, in your social environment. When you slow down your eating routine, you can begin to listen to what needs attention in your life and then look for alternative ways to cope with what's stressful.

It's important to find other things in life besides food that bring you pleasure, and this involves taking risks to try out new activities as well as new ways of relating to people and oneself. Some people find it helps if they don't schedule social engagements that revolve around food. This can be challenging for busy people who like to meet for meals and drinks to socialize.

Finding these alternative ways beyond food to self-soothe may not initially deliver as much pleasure as a doughnut, but it's important to realize that using other skills to manage feelings will provide some relief. If you're someone who uses food to cope with things, not being able to grab for a cookie can make you start to feel very anxious. It's difficult, but what you need to do is really sit with the emotions. Breathe, pause, stay with it, and realize that this is a time to make a mini-decision.

Watch what comes up mentally or physically as a result of breaking your routine. This will point to what parts of you or your environment need attention and perhaps some action or change.

What were the usual reasons you would override your hunger, Randy? Was it emotional?

RJ: For me it was basically the way I grew up. In the South your life revolves around family, work, and eating. I love Louisiana, but thank God I got out and wound up in California, which is more health conscious! But I had to retrain myself so I wasn't always eating "like a house on fire" as they say down there. I'm a pretty happy guy, but I used to constantly augment that happiness with food. Let's get doubly happy! I don't do that anymore.

Dr. Locker: That's an important point. There are a lot of ads out there that say, if you eat this food, you will be happy if you're sad and happier if you're already happy. But it doesn't work in the long run.

RJ: By the same token, losing weight might not make you happy either.

Dr. Locker: I often hear people say, "I'll start my life when I lose weight." "If I lose twenty pounds, I'll start to date, and then I'll be happy." They put their life on hold, waiting to lose weight. But even if you do lose weight you are still stuck with yourself and your same vulnerabilities. It's actually when you get a fuller, more authentic life through accepting what makes you like and dislike yourself that you feel happier and *that* helps you have success at sticking to healthy eating and exercise. If you work on accepting parts of yourself before you even begin trying to lose weight, or as you're going through the process, you're more likely to achieve long-term success.

RJ: What do you think is the best advice for someone who really needs to get a food divorce?

Dr. Locker: First, get clear on whether food is effective in making you feel better. So if you say, "I really want a piece of pie," you need to ask yourself, "What do I think it's going to do for me? Well, if I eat the pie, I'll feel less stressed and I'll feel a little bit of a sugar rush, and that might just make me feel better enough to get through the day." Okay, fine, so eat the pie. But then afterward you need to ask yourself, "Did it do what I thought it would do? Did it really fulfill that deep longing that I had to be with my soul mate or to have more vacation in my life? No, I felt great for about two minutes. It was great to eat it, but it didn't really make the profound change that I thought it would."

It's typical to think, "I'll feel so much better once I've had that dessert or once I have that great dinner," and then realize that it doesn't make any lasting changes in your mood. It's also typical to eventually find that the food doesn't hold its magic anymore. You may continue to eat it out of habit, but after a while it doesn't even register in taking away the stress or increasing the joy. Did you ever feel disappointed after a big meal?

RJ: Sometimes. Believe me, I enjoy a good meal, but food can only do so much for you. And I think that if you're using food to help you cope, it can really only provide you with momentary relief and, ultimately, a false sense of happiness. You're lying to yourself if you think it provides more. So my thing is, stop the lying. Look at yourself in the mirror and ask, "Why am I eating all this food? Let me figure out a way to get off this crazy food cycle that I'm on. Because it's not going to make me happy and it might even kill me."

I should distinguish between food making you a happy person and food giving you pleasure. I don't believe in denying yourself foods that give you pleasure. Make a rule for yourself that you're not going to have any chocolate and you know what? Eventually you're going to have that chocolate.

Dr. Locker: Yes. So say it's your birthday and you want a cupcake. Consciously and "mindfully" eat the cupcake and enjoy it. By "mindfully" I mean eating when you are hungry and stopping when you are full, based on your stomach sensations as well as paying attention to the sensory experiences of chewing the cupcake beyond just taste. Get into it. But don't have that cupcake be the *only* thing that makes you happy. That's when it becomes a problem.

RJ: Before I finally changed my eating and exercise habits for good, I stopped and started a million diets. I finally realized that I had to have patience and not go for the quick fix, but it's hard for a lot of people to be patient. What do you think can help people stay motivated?

Dr. Locker: One thing I think people can do is visualize and then write down what they'd like their life to be like if they weren't always struggling with food and exercise. It can help to have an awareness of the meaningful reasons for sticking with a challenging process. It could be something like, "Maybe I could go to the beach one day and not wear a huge drapey dress." Or, "Maybe I want to be able to walk into the Gap and not feel embarrassed."

RJ: Yeah, instead of going to Rochester Big & Tall or Lane Bryant. Who doesn't want to be able to shop at regular stores?

Dr. Locker: If you have made a list of reasons, you can go back and consult that list as to why you're trying to lose weight in the first place. That's a good way to remind yourself of why you need to keep going when the going gets tough.

RJ: I also think it's important to have realistic goals. Ten pounds: start there then see where you can go. What about weighing yourself? Do you think that's a good idea?

Dr. Locker: I'm not a fan of the scale because it's easy to become obsessed with it. The number on the scale can determine if you have a good or a bad day. If it goes up, it can trigger feelings of, "Well, fine, I might as well throw in the towel and just keep eating."

RJ: Then there are those times when you hit a plateau and you don't lose a pound for a few weeks so you think, "Okay, forget it, this thing is over." But of course it's not. There are always going to be setbacks.

Dr. Locker: Slow and steady wins the race. It's worthwhile to aim for having a "life worth living" where you aren't so tormented by food and constant questions: "What did I eat?" "What am I going to eat next?" And so on. It helps to become clear on how much of your emotional life is spent worrying about food and weight, then to work to break free of being the gerbil on the wheel of food obsession.

Another thing I believe helps people stay motivated is eating mindfully, which I mentioned earlier. The awareness of eating when you're hungry and stopping when you're full is a way of getting in touch with your body, and there is a kind of spiritual element to it because you're more attuned to how your body and mind affect each other. It gives you the feeling that your body is not just a separate vehicle that's walking you through life. Your body gives you signals, then you respond to them and body and mind become more integrated. This provides an opportunity to find ways to take care of those signals instead of overriding them, and so the spiritual aspect of heightened self-awareness and compassionate self-care comes into play.

RJ: Earlier in our conversation you said that if you don't work on the inside, the only thing that changes about you when you lose weight is your physical size. I think that's true. Here's the thing: people often treat you differently. That's what I found when I lost a lot of weight on a liquid diet. And not only did people treat me differently, I didn't like how I looked or felt. It was confusing.

Dr. Locker: When someone says to you, "God, Randy, you look fabulous," it's hard not to feel like, "Well, what did you think of me before?" I think it's really up to you to set the boundaries around comments related to your body. It's not really their business. If you do not want to discuss your weight, then change the subject.

It's also important to figure out what body size is really right for you. A lot of women say they want to be a size zero because it's fashionable. Well, a size zero is not only drastic, it is unrealistic and unhealthy for most people.

One of the main motivating factors for many people trying to lose weight, particularly when it comes to exercise, is that they want to look better. If you're going to be honest, that's a motivator. And there's nothing wrong with that as long as you know what's realistic for you and you are able to define yourself beyond how you look.

RJ: Everyone can't be the same size. It has to be a weight that's really going to work for you and that you're going to be able to accept.

Dr. Locker: And a weight that's healthy not only physically but also emotionally, right?

RJ: Right!

I have learned a lot in the last few years. A lot about how to get your life back on track when diagnosed with a frightening disease. A lot about why quick-fix diets don't work. And, most important, a lot about myself. I wish I didn't have to go to such drastic measures—having a gastric bypass—to get this great education, but I'm glad I did.

In some ways what that surgery did was help me flip the switch, taking me from someone struggling to eat healthfully and exercise regularly to someone who now has healthy habits. Let me draw up one final *Idol* metaphor to explain the switch premise. Over the years there have been contestants—I think you might know who I mean—who had incredible raw talent, but they just couldn't take it to the next level. For whatever reason, maybe it was that they were unable to perform their best under pressure or that they hadn't yet figured out what kind of artist they wanted to be, they could not find their footing and flip that switch. Yet some of them eventually did, and they went on to have success. They learned about themselves and, finally, something clicked.

That's essentially what happened to me in my battle to change my eating and exercise habits. When I look back at my weight-loss efforts before my diagnosis and surgery, one thing I now realize is that perfectionism was often my undoing. If I couldn't stay 100 percent on a program, I considered myself off that program. That was it. I was finished. What I've learned now—and not just as it relates to eating but as it relates to other aspects of my life, including tennis and music—is that you never want to hang on to a bad moment. When I succumb to a plate of syrup-drenched pancakes or lose a tennis match or have a bad session in the studio, I can't let that moment ruin the rest of my day.

So, okay, you fell off the wagon and ate twelve grilled cheese sandwiches. Guess what? There's still eight hours of daylight left. Try to correct it. Don't get caught up in that moment. "Oh hell, I blew it, let me continue to blow it all day.

Bring on the coconut cookies." Don't let one bad decision ruin your whole day, week, or life. "A slip doesn't equal a slide," says Dr. Locker. "Instead of saying, 'I'll start again on Monday,' turn it around at the next meal or snack. Get back on track. Let go of the past, even if it's earlier that very day, and focus on the present. Use the very moment you're in and the food choices before you in that present moment to make a healthy mini-decision."

These days, that's a rule I live by. If I'm not perfect, so what? I know I'm doing pretty well. I know, too, that I'm not and will never be the skinniest guy onstage, but I feel as though my body is just where I want it to be: strong, healthy, and in remission from diabetes. That makes me happy in a way that no cinnamon roll or chocolate bar ever could. And besides, you can be hot at any healthy size; see it in yourself and others will see it too.

Superstars cross my path every week, and I know that they're not perfect. But they know how to turn their negatives into positives. They know that it's your talents that matter, whether your talent is having an amazing voice or being an amazing friend to someone or being a great parent or being excellent at your job. I could go on and on because there are so many different things that people are good at. When you see and appreciate the talent in yourself, that's when you'll shine. That's when you'll flip the switch.

As I said in the beginning of this book, there is nothing more important when it comes to achieving your goal of good health than believing in yourself and being in touch with who you are. Whether you're a singer or a transit worker, an actor or a teacher, a writer or an accountant, you've got to learn to deal with your own stuff. Stay in your own lane. Don't worry about Bob or Sally. Figure out what works for you and stick with it.

And find what you love to do. It's funny, but something that I think can really help anyone reach the goal of achieving a healthy weight and giving up dieting forever is to be absolutely passionate about something (other than food, of course). When you are engaged in an activity that you love—and it could be anything from playing the piano to reading spy novels to crafting pottery to taking care of your kids—it takes your focus off eating. True, you have to find a balance. You don't want to forget all about eating, because that's when you're going to go too long without it and make yourself susceptible to overeating. That, as I've recounted, was my big mistake. I could get into that nothing-else-exists zone for hours when playing music, but I always let it go too far. Now I've got it under control, not only when I'm in the studio, but when I'm putting in those ten- to twelve-hour days during the initial *American Idol* auditions. So that's key, and if you can get that right, then I do think there is something to be said for finding something you can give yourself over to. That's known as the "I found my passion" weight-loss plan.

In the final analysis, I see myself as a living example of what does and doesn't work. Diets don't work. Eating better, eating less, moving, and having a positive attitude does. It's also so important to remember that this is a lifelong journey. It's not a sprint; it's not for two months; it's not to get you ready for the beach or for a wedding. When weight is your Achilles' heel, it's a lifelong struggle. Let's join together and get on with it. This is your mission—choose to accept it.

ACKNOWLEDGMENTS

I am a lucky man—lucky because after a close call I am again in good health. And lucky because I am blessed with the love and support of an incredible network of family, friends, and colleagues, including many who contributed to the creation of this book.

I am grateful first and foremost to my amazing wife, Erika, and equally amazing kids, Taylor, Zoe, and Jordan. Many thanks to Daryn Eller for all her hard work on this project, and to her family for putting up with all this nonsense! My managers Harriet Sternberg and Abe Hoch, Holly Boynton, Kenny Edwards, and everyone else at Dream Merchant 21 Entertainment have been indispensable. You guys are the greatest.

Thanks to agents Richard Pine and Elisa Petrini at InkWell Management for easing me through the publishing process, and to Luke Dempsey, Clare Ferraro, Marie Coolman, Liz Keenan, and Danielle Friedman at Hudson Street Press for their editorial guiding hands.

Acknowledgments

When I needed expertise, I went to the experts and they delivered in great measure. A big thanks to Erin Naimi, RD, Janeen Locker, PhD, Jeff Parker, Tarik Tyler, Brittania Erickson, and Catherine Chiarelli.

For medical expertise, inspiration, and support, I am grateful to Frances Kaufman, MD, Mal Fobi, MD, Dan Jones, MD, president of the American Heart Association, and Takeda Pharmaceuticals.

I get inspiration, too, from a few other people working tirelessly to help others. Thanks to Oprah for continuing to use your show to enlighten and motivate people to lead healthier lives, and to Mark Shriver at Save the Children, for all the programs and initiatives you work on to better the lives of kids around the world.

I also want to express my appreciation to all those people who make my life and work a little easier and a lot more fun: Lee Phillips, Ed Astrin, Kelli Barton, Tracy Gray at Nike, everyone at MTV's *America's Best Dance Crew*, Fox, 19 Entertainment, FremantleMedia, film and TV agent Sean Perry at Endeavor, and music agent Jeff Frasco at CAA. Not to mention Paula Abdul, Ryan Seacrest, and Simon Cowell. To my brother, Herman Jackson Jr., and sister, Sue Ann Lewis, thanks for helping make some of the memories recounted on these pages. And props to Clay Patrick McBride for the dope picture on the cover.

Finally, for all the blessings of this crazy life I love, I thank God.